I0698326

Optimizing Life With Osteoarthritis

Optimizing Life With Osteoarthritis

Strategies for pain management and quality living

Victor Asher

Dedication

This book is dedicated to God All-Powerful for His grace and wisdom, to my family, to my beautiful readers who will find this book relevant to them, and to everyone who has loved, supported, and encouraged me along the way. I would not be in the position I am in today without your unshakable faith in me. I dedicate this book to all my readers especially those with bone issues and pray this to be of help to you all.

Contents

Acknowledgement

I want to sincerely thank God for providing the means and insight that guided me during the writing of this book. I cannot forget my family members, whose encouragement and support have given me bravery and motivation throughout the process.

Thank you to my editor and publisher for their crucial advice and help in bringing this project to its successful conclusion. I would like to express my gratitude to everyone who so kindly contributed their time and knowledge to this project and added their wisdom. I want to express my gratitude to my friends as well, I appreciate all of your steadfast love and support throughout the journey. Finally, I extend my thanks to each and every one of you for purchasing and reading my work. I am thankful it met your needs and added to your knowledge. I sincerely value each and every one of you and think you're all fantastic.

Introduction

Osteoarthritis, often referred to as the "wear and tear" arthritis, affects millions of people around the world. It is a chronic condition that primarily affects the joints, causing pain, stiffness, and reduced mobility. While it is most commonly associated with aging, osteoarthritis can also develop as a result of joint injuries, obesity, genetic factors, and other underlying conditions.

The journey of living with osteoarthritis can be challenging and daunting, as the pain and limitations it imposes can significantly impact one's quality of life. However, it is important to remember that there is hope and that there are numerous strategies and treatments available to manage the symptoms and enhance your overall well-being.

This book, "Living with Osteoarthritis: Managing Pain and Enhancing Quality of Life," is designed to be your comprehensive guide through the maze of osteoarthritis management. Whether you have recently been diagnosed with osteoarthritis or have been living with it for years, this book aims to empower you with knowledge, tools, and practical advice to navigate the complexities of this condition and regain control over your life.

In the following pages, we will explore various aspects of osteoarthritis, from understanding its causes and risk factors to diagnosing the condition accurately. We will delve into the different treatment options available, including both conventional and alternative approaches, providing you with valuable insights to make informed decisions about your care.

Moreover, this book recognizes the importance of a holistic approach to managing osteoarthritis. It addresses not only physical pain management but also emotional well-being, lifestyle modifications, and supportive strategies to enhance your overall quality of life. By adopting a multidimensional approach, we can better address the challenges posed by osteoarthritis and work towards improving your day-to-day experiences.

Furthermore, we understand the significance of self-empowerment and self-care in the face of osteoarthritis. You will find practical advice on creating personalized exercise routines, implementing joint protection techniques, and adopting a nourishing diet that supports joint health. Additionally, we will explore the role of assistive devices, complementary therapies, and surgical options for advanced cases, ensuring you have a comprehensive understanding of the available resources and treatments.

Living with osteoarthritis is a journey that requires resilience, adaptability, and a proactive mindset. By equipping yourself with knowledge and embracing the strategies outlined in this book, you can take charge of your osteoarthritis management, alleviate pain, and enhance your overall quality of life. Remember, you are not alone on this journey. There is a vast community of individuals experiencing similar challenges, and through shared experiences and support, we can inspire each other to lead fulfilling lives despite the presence of osteoarthritis.

Now, let us embark on this empowering journey together, discovering the tools and strategies that will enable you to live a life that is not defined by osteoarthritis, but rather, enriched by resilience, self-care, and a renewed sense of well-being.

Chapter 1

Understanding Osteoarthritis

What is Osteoarthritis?

Osteoarthritis is a degenerative joint disease characterized by the breakdown and gradual loss of cartilage in the joints. It is the most common form of arthritis and primarily affects the weight-bearing joints such as the knees, hips, and spine, as well as the hands and fingers. The progressive loss of cartilage leads to joint pain, stiffness, swelling, and reduced range of motion. Osteoarthritis often develops slowly and worsens over time, impacting a person's ability to perform daily activities and leading to decreased quality of life.

Historical Perspective

Osteoarthritis has been a part of human history for centuries, although the understanding and recognition of the condition have evolved over time. Here is a brief overview of the history of osteoarthritis:

- **Ancient Times**

Evidence of osteoarthritis has been found in ancient human remains, providing insight into the presence of the condition in prehistoric populations. Archaeological studies have revealed signs of osteoarthritis in skeletal remains dating back thousands of years, indicating that the disease has affected humans for a long time.

- **18th and 19th Centuries**

During the 18th and 19th centuries, physicians and scientists began to recognize and describe osteoarthritis. In 1804, Jean-Martin Charcot, a French physician, coined the term "osteoarthritis" to distinguish it from other forms of arthritis, such as rheumatoid arthritis. Charcot's work laid the foundation for understanding the distinct characteristics and features of osteoarthritis.

- **20th Century**

In the early 20th century, advancements in radiology allowed for better visualization of joint changes associated with osteoarthritis. X-ray technology enabled physicians to observe joint space narrowing, the formation of osteophytes (bone spurs), and other structural changes that occur in osteoarthritis. These findings contributed to improved diagnosis and understanding of the disease.

Later in the 20th century, research and medical advancements furthered our knowledge of osteoarthritis. Studies focused on the mechanisms underlying cartilage degradation, the role of inflammation in the disease process, and the genetic and environmental factors influencing its development. This period also saw the development of various treatment options, including medications, physical therapy, and surgical interventions.

- **21st Century**

In recent decades, there has been a growing emphasis on patient-centered care and holistic management of osteoarthritis. The importance of lifestyle modifications, exercise, weight management, and self-care in reducing symptoms and improving quality of life has gained recognition. Research continues to explore new therapies, regenerative medicine approaches, and personalized treatment options for osteoarthritis.

The understanding and management of osteoarthritis have significantly evolved throughout history. Today, it is recognized as a common and complex joint disease that requires a multidisciplinary approach, involving healthcare professionals, patients, and researchers working together to advance knowledge and improve outcomes for individuals living with osteoarthritis.

Causes and Risk Factors

Osteoarthritis, a complex condition, can be influenced by various causes and risk factors. While the precise cause is not fully understood, the following factors contribute to the development and progression of osteoarthritis:

1. Age

Age is a significant risk factor for the development of osteoarthritis. As individuals grow older, the risk of developing the condition increases. Cartilage, which acts as a protective cushion between the bones in the joints, naturally undergoes wear and tear over time. This normal aging process can lead to the gradual degeneration of cartilage, making it more susceptible to damage and contributing to the development of osteoarthritis.

With age, the ability of cartilage to repair and regenerate itself decreases, resulting in a loss of its structural integrity. The cartilage becomes thinner and less capable of absorbing the forces and impact placed on the joints during movement. As a result, the joint surfaces may experience increased friction, leading to the breakdown of cartilage and the development of osteoarthritis.

Furthermore, aging is often accompanied by other factors that can contribute to the development of osteoarthritis. These factors include a decrease in muscle strength and flexibility, changes in hormone levels, and the presence of other age-related health conditions. Additionally, lifestyle factors such as sedentary behavior, poor nutrition, and obesity, which can become more prevalent with age, can further exacerbate the risk of developing osteoarthritis.

While age is a significant risk factor for osteoarthritis, it is important to note that not everyone will develop the condition solely based on age. There are individuals who maintain healthy joints well into old age, while others may experience osteoarthritis at a younger age due to other contributing factors. Nonetheless, understanding the impact of age on joint health and taking proactive measures to maintain joint function and overall health can play a crucial role in reducing the risk and managing osteoarthritis effectively.

2. Joint Trauma or Injury

Previous joint injuries, such as fractures, ligament Joint trauma or injury is a significant risk factor for the development of osteoarthritis. Previous injuries to the joints, such as fractures, ligament tears, or repetitive stress injuries, can increase the likelihood of developing osteoarthritis in the affected joint.

When a joint undergoes trauma or injury, it can disrupt the normal structure and function of the joint. The initial damage to the joint can lead to an inflammatory response, causing the release of certain enzymes and substances that can accelerate the breakdown of cartilage. The inflammatory process, if not properly resolved, can contribute to the ongoing degeneration of cartilage and the development of osteoarthritis.

Fractures that involve the joint surface, ligament injuries that result in joint instability, or repetitive stress injuries that repeatedly strain the joint can all contribute to the increased risk of osteoarthritis. These injuries can cause mechanical abnormalities within the joint, alter joint mechanics, and create uneven forces on the cartilage. Over time, this increased stress and abnormal load distribution can accelerate the breakdown of cartilage and promote the onset of osteoarthritis.

It is important to note that not all joint injuries will lead to osteoarthritis. The severity and type of injury, the location of the injury, and individual factors such as age, genetics, and overall joint health can all influence the risk of developing osteoarthritis following joint trauma or injury.

Taking prompt and appropriate measures to treat and rehabilitate joint injuries, including physical therapy, exercises, and protective measures, can help reduce the risk of developing osteoarthritis. Additionally, maintaining overall joint health through regular exercise, weight management, and proper joint mechanics can play a role in minimizing the long-term impact of joint injuries and reducing the risk of osteoarthritis.

3. Genetics

Genetic factors indeed play a role in the susceptibility to osteoarthritis. Certain gene variations can influence the development and progression of the condition by affecting various aspects of joint health, including cartilage metabolism, joint stability, and inflammation.

- **Cartilage Metabolism**

Genes involved in the regulation of cartilage metabolism, such as those encoding enzymes responsible for collagen synthesis and degradation, can influence the integrity and resilience of cartilage. Variations in these genes may lead to an imbalance in cartilage turnover, resulting in accelerated cartilage breakdown and the development of osteoarthritis.

- **Joint Stability**

Genes involved in joint development, structure, and stability can impact the risk of osteoarthritis. Variations in genes responsible for ligament and tendon integrity, joint alignment, and joint capsule function can affect the stability of the joint. Instability or improper alignment of the joint can increase the mechanical stress on the cartilage, leading to its degeneration and the onset of osteoarthritis.

- **Inflammation**

Inflammatory processes play a role in the development and progression of osteoarthritis. Genes involved in regulating the immune response and inflammation can influence the risk of developing the condition. Variations in these genes may contribute to an imbalance in inflammatory factors, leading to chronic low-grade inflammation within the joint and the subsequent breakdown of cartilage.

It is important to note that genetics alone do not determine whether an individual will develop osteoarthritis. The interplay between genetic factors and environmental or lifestyle factors is crucial in understanding disease susceptibility. Environmental factors, such as joint trauma, obesity, and occupation, can further interact with genetic predispositions to influence the development of osteoarthritis.

While it is not currently possible to alter one's genetic makeup, understanding the role of genetic factors in osteoarthritis can help identify individuals at higher risk. This knowledge can aid in implementing proactive strategies for joint health, such as regular exercise, weight management, and lifestyle modifications, to minimize the impact of genetic predisposition and potentially delay the onset or progression of osteoarthritis.

4. Obesity

Obesity is a significant risk factor for the development and progression of osteoarthritis. Excessive body weight places additional stress on weight-bearing joints, such as the knees and hips, which can have detrimental effects on joint health.

The mechanical stress caused by excess weight puts a greater load on the joints, particularly during weight-bearing activities such as walking or running. This increased load can lead to increased wear and tear on the cartilage, which serves as a protective cushion between the bones in the joint. Over time, the continuous pressure and strain can contribute to cartilage damage and accelerate the progression of osteoarthritis.

In addition to the direct mechanical impact, obesity can also promote a state of chronic low-grade inflammation in the body. Fat cells, especially those located in and around the joints, release inflammatory substances known as cytokines. These cytokines can trigger an inflammatory response within the joint, further contributing to cartilage breakdown and the development of osteoarthritis.

Weight distribution and body mechanics also play a role in the impact of obesity on joint health. Excess weight can lead to altered joint alignment and increased stress on specific areas of the joint, exacerbating the risk of osteoarthritis development. For example, in the knee joint, obesity can lead to a misalignment of forces, resulting in uneven wear on the cartilage surfaces.

It is important to recognize that obesity not only increases the risk of developing osteoarthritis but can also worsen the symptoms and progression of existing osteoarthritis. Therefore, weight management and maintaining a healthy body weight are crucial in the prevention and management of osteoarthritis.

By maintaining a healthy weight through a combination of regular physical activity, a balanced diet, and lifestyle modifications, individuals can reduce the mechanical stress on their joints and decrease the risk of developing osteoarthritis. Weight loss in individuals who are already overweight or obese can also provide symptomatic relief and improve the overall management of osteoarthritis.

5. Joint Alignment and Structure

Joint alignment and structure play a crucial role in joint health and can impact the risk of developing osteoarthritis. Abnormalities in joint alignment, misalignments, or congenital conditions can disrupt the normal distribution of forces within the joint, leading to increased wear and tear on specific areas.

In a healthy joint, the forces and loads generated during movement are evenly distributed across the joint surfaces and the surrounding structures, such as cartilage and ligaments. This balanced distribution of forces helps to maintain the integrity and function of the joint. However, when there are abnormalities in joint alignment or structure, the forces may be concentrated on certain areas, resulting in increased stress and accelerated wear and tear on those regions.

Misalignments can occur due to various reasons, such as joint injuries, previous fractures, or developmental abnormalities. For example, conditions like bowed legs or unequal leg length can cause uneven weight distribution on the joints, leading to excessive stress on specific areas. Similarly, joint abnormalities or congenital conditions like hip dysplasia can result in improper joint alignment and instability, predisposing the joint to increased wear and tear.

The uneven distribution of forces within the joint can cause localized damage to the cartilage, leading to its breakdown over time. As the cartilage wears away, the underlying bone may become exposed and vulnerable, leading to further joint degeneration and the development of osteoarthritis.

It is important to note that joint alignment and structure can be influenced by a combination of genetic and environmental factors. While some individuals may be born with certain joint abnormalities, others may develop them as a result of injuries, overuse, or lifestyle factors. By addressing these alignment issues and seeking appropriate medical interventions, such as physical therapy, orthopedic devices, or surgical procedures, individuals can help restore proper joint mechanics and reduce the risk of osteoarthritis.

Additionally, maintaining overall joint health through exercises that promote strength, stability, and flexibility can be beneficial in managing the impact of joint alignment and structure on osteoarthritis risk. Strengthening the muscles surrounding the joints can help provide better support and stability, potentially mitigating the excessive stress on specific areas of the joint.

In summary, joint abnormalities, misalignments, or congenital conditions can contribute to the uneven distribution of forces on the joints, leading to increased wear and tear on specific areas. Understanding and addressing these alignment issues can play a crucial role in reducing the risk of osteoarthritis and maintaining joint health.

6. Gender

Gender differences play a role in the prevalence and distribution of osteoarthritis. Osteoarthritis is more common in women, with certain joints, such as the hands and knees, being particularly affected. While the exact reasons for this gender disparity are not fully understood, several factors contribute to this observation.

Hormonal factors have been proposed as one potential explanation. Hormones, such as estrogen, play a role in maintaining joint health and regulating inflammation. During menopause, when estrogen levels decline, women may experience changes in joint structure and mechanics, leading to an increased risk of osteoarthritis. The decline in estrogen levels can also contribute to the loss of cartilage resilience and the overall integrity of the joints.

Differences in joint structure and mechanics between men and women may also contribute to the gender disparity in osteoarthritis. Women generally have a different joint anatomy, including narrower joint spaces and smaller articular surfaces, compared to men. These structural differences may increase the susceptibility of women to certain types of joint degeneration and osteoarthritis.

Furthermore, lifestyle and occupational factors may also contribute to the higher prevalence of osteoarthritis in women. Women often engage in activities or occupations that involve repetitive movements or prolonged periods of joint stress, which can contribute to joint wear and tear. Additionally, women may have higher rates of obesity, which further increases the mechanical stress on weight-bearing joints.

It is important to note that while osteoarthritis is more common in women, men are still at risk of developing the condition, especially in joints such as the hips or spine. The gender disparity in osteoarthritis highlights the need for considering gender-specific factors in prevention, diagnosis, and treatment approaches.

By understanding the impact of gender on osteoarthritis, healthcare professionals can provide tailored care, including appropriate management strategies and interventions, to address the specific needs of women and men. Additionally, promoting joint health through regular exercise, weight management, and lifestyle modifications can be beneficial for both genders in reducing the risk and managing osteoarthritis effectively.

7. Occupation and Activities

Occupation and activities can have a significant impact on joint health and increase the risk of developing osteoarthritis. Certain occupations and activities that involve repetitive joint movements, heavy lifting, or prolonged kneeling can subject the joints to increased stress and contribute to joint damage over time.

- **Repetitive joint movements**

Occupations or activities that require repetitive joint movements, such as assembly line work, typing, or playing certain musical instruments, can increase the risk of developing osteoarthritis. Continuous and repetitive motions can lead to the breakdown of cartilage and cause excessive wear and tear on the joints involved. Over time, this repetitive stress can contribute to the development of osteoarthritis.

- **Heavy lifting**

Jobs or activities that involve heavy lifting, such as construction work or manual labor, can put significant strain on the joints, particularly those in the back, shoulders, and knees. The excessive load placed on the joints can lead to joint damage and accelerate the progression of osteoarthritis. Improper lifting techniques or inadequate support and protection for the joints can further increase the risk.

- **Prolonged kneeling**

Occupations or activities that require prolonged kneeling, such as flooring installation, gardening, or plumbing, can increase the risk of developing osteoarthritis in the knees. Prolonged pressure and stress on the knee joints while in a kneeling position can cause cartilage breakdown and joint inflammation, contributing to the development of osteoarthritis.

It is important to note that not all individuals exposed to these occupational or activity-related factors will develop osteoarthritis. The risk may depend on several factors, including the duration and intensity of the exposure, individual susceptibility, joint health, and the presence of other risk factors.

Taking preventive measures can help reduce the risk of joint damage and osteoarthritis in these situations. This may include implementing proper ergonomics and joint protection techniques, taking regular breaks to rest and stretch, using assistive devices or equipment to minimize joint stress, and engaging in exercises that promote joint strength and flexibility. Additionally, workplace modifications and occupational safety measures can be implemented to reduce the impact of occupational factors on joint health.

If you are engaged in an occupation or activity that involves repetitive joint movements, heavy lifting, or prolonged kneeling, it is advisable to consult with a healthcare professional or occupational therapist to develop strategies to protect your joints and minimize the risk of developing osteoarthritis.

8. Medical Conditions

Having certain medical conditions can increase the risk of developing osteoarthritis. Conditions such as rheumatoid arthritis, gout, and metabolic disorders can predispose individuals to the development of osteoarthritis.

- **Rheumatoid arthritis**

Rheumatoid arthritis is an autoimmune disease characterized by chronic joint inflammation. The inflammation associated with rheumatoid arthritis can damage the cartilage and lead to joint erosion. Over time, this joint damage can contribute to the development of secondary osteoarthritis. Individuals with rheumatoid arthritis are at an increased risk of developing osteoarthritis, particularly in the affected joints.

- **Gout**

Gout is a type of arthritis caused by the buildup of uric acid crystals in the joints. Chronic gout can lead to joint damage and inflammation, which can contribute to the development of osteoarthritis. The presence of gout increases the risk of developing secondary osteoarthritis, especially in the joints affected by gout attacks.

- **Metabolic disorders**

Metabolic disorders such as diabetes, obesity, and metabolic syndrome have been associated with an increased risk of developing osteoarthritis. These conditions can contribute to systemic inflammation, insulin resistance, and alterations in metabolic processes, which may promote cartilage degeneration and the development of osteoarthritis.

It's important to note that the relationship between these medical conditions and osteoarthritis is complex and multifactorial. The mechanisms linking these conditions to osteoarthritis development are still being researched, and there may be additional factors involved.

If you have any of these medical conditions, it is important to work closely with your healthcare provider to manage and control the underlying condition. This may involve appropriate medical treatments, lifestyle modifications, and regular monitoring. By effectively managing these conditions, you may be able to reduce the risk or slow down the progression of osteoarthritis.

Additionally, maintaining a healthy lifestyle, including regular exercise, weight management, and a balanced diet, can help support joint health and reduce the impact of these medical conditions on the development of osteoarthritis.

9. Joint Inflammation

Chronic joint inflammation can have a significant impact on the development and progression of osteoarthritis. Whether caused by previous joint injury, underlying conditions, or systemic inflammation, it can contribute to cartilage breakdown and accelerate the progression of osteoarthritis.

Inflammation is the body's natural response to injury, infection, or other harmful stimuli. It involves the activation of the immune system and the release of various inflammatory substances, such as cytokines and enzymes. While acute inflammation is a protective response aimed at healing and repair, chronic inflammation can be detrimental to joint health.

- **Previous joint injury**

A previous joint injury, such as a fracture, ligament tear, or meniscus tear, can lead to chronic inflammation in the affected joint. The ongoing inflammatory response can disrupt the normal functioning of the joint and contribute to the breakdown of cartilage over time. The damaged or inflamed tissues release substances that can further promote inflammation and contribute to the development of osteoarthritis.

- **Underlying conditions**

Certain underlying conditions, such as rheumatoid arthritis, psoriatic arthritis, or lupus, are characterized by chronic joint inflammation. These conditions involve an abnormal immune response that targets the joints, leading to persistent inflammation. The chronic inflammation in these conditions can damage the cartilage, leading to joint deterioration and the development of secondary osteoarthritis.

- **Systemic inflammation**

Systemic inflammation, which can occur due to factors such as obesity, metabolic syndrome, or chronic low-grade infections, can also contribute to the progression of osteoarthritis. Systemic inflammation affects the entire body, including the joints. The inflammatory substances released during systemic inflammation can directly impact the cartilage and accelerate its breakdown, leading to the development or worsening of osteoarthritis.

The inflammatory processes associated with chronic joint inflammation can cause the release of enzymes that degrade the cartilage matrix, leading to cartilage damage and loss. Additionally, chronic inflammation can disrupt the balance between cartilage synthesis and degradation, favoring the breakdown of cartilage.

Managing chronic joint inflammation is important in reducing the risk and slowing down the progression of osteoarthritis. This may involve appropriate medical treatments, such as anti-inflammatory medications or disease-modifying drugs, as well as lifestyle modifications to reduce inflammation, such as regular exercise, stress management, and a healthy diet.

It is essential for individuals with chronic joint inflammation to work closely with their healthcare providers to develop a comprehensive treatment plan that addresses both the underlying condition and the management of osteoarthritis risk. By effectively managing inflammation, it is possible to minimize its impact on cartilage health and promote better joint outcomes.

10. Joint Overuse

Joint overuse is a significant risk factor for the development of osteoarthritis. Excessive and repetitive use of joints, particularly in activities or sports that involve repetitive impact of stress on the joints, can contribute to the breakdown of cartilage and increase the likelihood of developing osteoarthritis.

When joints are subjected to repetitive movements or excessive loading, the cartilage that cushions the joint surfaces can undergo wear and tear. Over time, this can lead to the breakdown of cartilage, resulting in joint damage and the development of osteoarthritis. The repetitive impact of stress on the joints can cause microtrauma, inflammation, and an imbalance in the joint's ability to repair and regenerate the cartilage.

Activities and sports that involve repetitive joint movements or high-impact actions pose a greater risk for joint overuse and subsequent osteoarthritis.

Some examples include:

- **Running and jogging**

The repetitive impact on weight-bearing joints, such as the knees and hips, during running or jogging can contribute to cartilage breakdown over time.

- **Jumping and landing sports**

Sports like basketball, volleyball, and gymnastics involve frequent jumping and landing, which can place significant stress on the joints, particularly in the lower extremities.

- **Repetitive lifting or manual labor**

Occupations or activities that require repetitive lifting, carrying heavy loads, or performing manual labor can strain the joints, leading to increased wear and tear.

- **Certain occupations**

Jobs that involve repetitive joint movements, such as assembly line work or typing, can also contribute to joint overuse and increase the risk of developing osteoarthritis.

While engaging in these activities or sports doesn't guarantee the development of osteoarthritis, individuals who participate in them regularly and intensively are at a higher risk. Other factors, such as individual joint health, genetics, and the presence of other risk factors, can also influence the development of osteoarthritis.

To mitigate the risk of joint overuse and osteoarthritis, it is important to take appropriate measures:

- **Practice proper technique and form**

Ensure that you are using correct form and technique during activities and sports to minimize excessive stress on the joints.

- **Gradual progression**

Gradually increase the intensity, duration, and frequency of activities or sports to allow the joints and tissues to adapt and strengthen over time.

- **Cross-training and variety**

Engage in a variety of activities and sports to avoid overloading specific joints and to promote overall joint health.

- **Adequate rest and recovery**

Allow sufficient time for rest and recovery between workouts or physical activities to give the joints time to repair and regenerate.

- **Joint protection**

Use appropriate protective equipment, such as knee pads or joint braces, when engaging in activities that involve increased joint stress.

By balancing physical activities, practicing proper technique, and incorporating rest and recovery, individuals can reduce the risk of joint overuse and help protect their joints from excessive wear and tear that can lead to osteoarthritis.

11. Hormonal Factors

Hormonal factors, particularly the changes that occur during menopause, can have an impact on joint health and contribute to the development of osteoarthritis in women. Menopause is a natural stage in a woman's life when her reproductive hormones, such as estrogen, decline.

Estrogen is known to have protective effects on joint health. It helps maintain the integrity of cartilage and has anti-inflammatory properties. Therefore, the decline in estrogen levels during menopause can potentially affect joint tissues and increase the risk of osteoarthritis. However, the exact mechanisms by which hormonal changes influence osteoarthritis are still being studied.

Here are some key points regarding the relationship between hormonal factors and osteoarthritis in women:

- **Menopause and estrogen decline**

During menopause, the ovaries gradually produce less estrogen, leading to a decrease in circulating estrogen levels. Estrogen plays a role in maintaining joint health by promoting the synthesis of collagen and proteoglycans, important components of cartilage. The decline in estrogen levels may disrupt this balance, making the joint tissues more susceptible to damage and contributing to the development of osteoarthritis.

- **Joint symptoms during menopause**

Some women may experience joint symptoms, such as pain, stiffness, or swelling, during or after menopause. These symptoms can be related to the hormonal changes occurring in the body. However, it's important to note that not all women experience joint symptoms during menopause, and the severity and prevalence of these symptoms can vary.

- **Localization of osteoarthritis in women**

Osteoarthritis commonly affects certain joints in women, such as the hands and knees. These joints may be more susceptible to hormonal influences, although the exact reasons for this localization are not fully understood. It's worth mentioning that osteoarthritis can affect other joints in both men and women as well.

- **Hormone replacement therapy (HRT)**

Hormone replacement therapy, which involves the use of estrogen or a combination of estrogen and progestin, is sometimes prescribed to manage menopausal symptoms. There has been ongoing research on the potential benefits and risks of HRT in relation to joint health and osteoarthritis. It's important for women considering HRT to discuss the potential benefits and risks with their healthcare providers, as HRT may have other effects on the body beyond joint health.

While hormonal factors, particularly the decline in estrogen levels during menopause, may contribute to the development of osteoarthritis in women, it's important to remember that osteoarthritis is a complex condition with multiple contributing factors. Other risk factors, such as age, genetics, obesity, joint overuse, and joint injuries, can also play significant roles in the development and progression of osteoarthritis.

If you are experiencing joint symptoms or have concerns about osteoarthritis related to hormonal changes, it is recommended to consult with your healthcare provider. They can provide personalized advice and guidance based on your individual circumstances and help manage any symptoms effectively.

12. Muscle Weakness and Imbalance

Muscle weakness and imbalance can play a role in the development of osteoarthritis. The muscles surrounding the joints provide support and stability, helping to distribute forces evenly during movement. When these muscles are weak or imbalanced, it can lead to increased stress on the joint structures, potentially contributing to the development of osteoarthritis.

Here are some key points regarding the relationship between muscle weakness, muscle imbalance, and osteoarthritis:

- **Muscle support for joint function**

Strong and balanced muscles play a crucial role in supporting joint function. They help absorb shock, stabilize the joints, and control movement. When muscles surrounding a joint are weak, the joint may be subjected to increased stress and impact during weight-bearing activities. This added stress can accelerate the wear and tear of cartilage and contribute to the development of osteoarthritis.

- **Joint alignment and muscle imbalances**

Muscles work in pairs or groups to move and stabilize the joints. When there is an imbalance in the strength or activation of these muscles, it can affect joint alignment and biomechanics. For example, if the muscles on one side of a joint are significantly weaker than the opposing muscles, it can lead to joint instability and abnormal forces on the joint surfaces. Over time, this can contribute to joint degeneration and the development of osteoarthritis.

- **Impact of muscle weakness on joint loading**

Weak muscles may not provide adequate support and shock absorption during physical activities. This can result in higher forces being transmitted to the joint structures, increasing the risk of cartilage damage and joint deterioration. Additionally, muscle weakness can affect joint movement patterns, leading to abnormal loading and uneven distribution of forces within the joint, further increasing the risk of osteoarthritis.

- **Rehabilitation and strengthening**

Addressing muscle weakness and imbalances through targeted exercises and rehabilitation can help improve joint stability, reduce stress on the joint structures, and potentially slow down the progression of osteoarthritis. Strengthening exercises that target the muscles surrounding the affected joint, as well as exercises that promote overall muscle balance and coordination, can be beneficial.

- **Comprehensive treatment approach**

Managing muscle weakness and imbalances should be part of a comprehensive treatment approach for osteoarthritis. This may include a combination of exercise therapy, physical therapy, and possibly assistance from healthcare professionals, such as physiotherapists or exercise specialists. These professionals can assess muscle imbalances, develop personalized exercise programs, and provide guidance on proper technique and progression.

It's important to note that muscle weakness and imbalance are not the sole causes of osteoarthritis, but they can contribute to joint deterioration and increase the risk of developing the condition. Adopting a proactive approach to strengthen and balance the muscles surrounding the joints can help improve joint stability, reduce stress on the joint structures, and potentially alleviate symptoms associated with osteoarthritis.

13. Certain Medications

Prolonged use of certain medications, particularly corticosteroids, has been associated with an increased risk of osteoarthritis. While medications are commonly used to manage various health conditions, it is important to be aware of the potential effects they may have on joint health.

Here are some key points regarding the relationship between certain medications and osteoarthritis:

- **Corticosteroids**

Corticosteroids are powerful anti-inflammatory medications that are commonly prescribed to reduce inflammation and manage symptoms in conditions such as rheumatoid arthritis, asthma, and other inflammatory disorders. However, prolonged use of corticosteroids, especially in higher doses, has been linked to an increased risk of osteoarthritis. These medications can affect the metabolism of cartilage and bone, leading to accelerated cartilage breakdown and potentially contributing to the development of osteoarthritis.

- **Other medications**

While corticosteroids are the medications most commonly associated with increased osteoarthritis risk, it is important to note that certain other medications may also have an impact. For example, some studies suggest that long-term use of certain anti-epileptic drugs and antibiotics may be associated with an increased risk of osteoarthritis, although further research is needed to establish clear causal relationships.

- **Balancing risks and benefits**

It is essential to weigh the potential risks and benefits of medications when considering their use. In many cases, the benefits of medications in managing underlying health conditions may outweigh the potential risks associated with osteoarthritis. It is important to have open and honest discussions with healthcare providers to understand the potential effects of medications on joint health and explore alternative treatment options if necessary.

- **Monitoring and management**

If you are on long-term medication use, particularly corticosteroids, it is important to have regular follow-up with your healthcare provider. They can monitor your joint health, assess for any signs of osteoarthritis, and provide appropriate management strategies to minimize the risk and impact of the condition. This may involve lifestyle modifications, exercise programs, and potential adjustments to medication regimens.

It's important to note that not everyone who takes medications, including corticosteroids, will develop osteoarthritis. The risk may vary depending on factors such as dosage, duration of use, and individual susceptibility. Additionally, the development of osteoarthritis is multifactorial, and other risk factors, such as age, genetics, and joint mechanics, also play significant roles.

If you have concerns about the potential effects of medications on your joint health or if you are experiencing joint symptoms, it is recommended to consult with your healthcare provider. They can provide personalized advice, evaluate your specific situation, and help guide you in managing your health condition while minimizing potential risks to joint health.

14. Environmental Factors

Environmental factors, including exposure to certain chemicals or toxins, have been suggested as possible contributors to the development of osteoarthritis. While the exact mechanisms are still being studied, there is evidence to suggest that environmental factors can play a role in the onset and progression of the condition.

Here are some key points regarding the relationship between environmental factors and osteoarthritis:

- **Occupational exposures**

Certain occupations that involve exposure to repetitive joint movements, vibrations, heavy lifting, or exposure to chemicals and toxins may increase the risk of developing osteoarthritis. For example, individuals working in jobs that require repetitive kneeling, squatting, or heavy lifting, such as construction workers or farmers, may be at higher risk. Additionally, exposure to hazardous substances like lead, asbestos, or certain solvents may contribute to the development of joint damage and osteoarthritis.

- **Environmental toxins**

Environmental factors, including air pollution and exposure to toxins, have also been implicated in the development of osteoarthritis. Studies have suggested a potential link between air pollutants, such as particulate matter, and the risk of developing osteoarthritis. These pollutants may have inflammatory effects on joint tissues, contributing to the degeneration of cartilage.

- **Joint inflammation and oxidative stress**

Environmental factors may induce joint inflammation and increase oxidative stress within the joints. This chronic inflammation and oxidative stress can lead to the breakdown of cartilage and the development of osteoarthritis. The specific mechanisms by which environmental factors contribute to joint inflammation and oxidative stress are still being investigated.

- **Individual susceptibility**

It's important to note that not everyone exposed to environmental factors will develop osteoarthritis. Individual susceptibility to these factors may vary, and the development of osteoarthritis is influenced by a combination of genetic, lifestyle, and environmental factors. While the relationship between environmental factors and osteoarthritis is still being explored, it is prudent to take steps to minimize exposure to potential hazards and maintain a healthy lifestyle.

Here are a few suggestions:

- Practice proper safety measures and use protective equipment in occupations or activities that involve repetitive joint movements, heavy lifting, or exposure to chemicals or toxins.
- Minimize exposure to environmental toxins and pollutants by following guidelines for air quality, avoiding smoking, and reducing exposure to hazardous substances.
- Adopt a healthy lifestyle that includes regular exercise, maintaining a balanced diet, managing weight, and avoiding behaviors that may increase the risk of joint damage.

If you have concerns about the potential impact of environmental factors on your joint health or if you are experiencing joint symptoms, it is advisable to consult with your healthcare provider. They can evaluate your individual circumstances, provide personalized advice, and help you make informed decisions to protect and maintain your joint health.

15. Inflammatory Joint Diseases

Chronic inflammatory joint diseases, such as rheumatoid arthritis (RA), can increase the risk of developing secondary osteoarthritis in the affected joints. While osteoarthritis and inflammatory joint diseases are distinct conditions, there can be an interplay between them.

Here are some key points regarding the relationship between inflammatory joint diseases and secondary osteoarthritis:

- **Joint inflammation and cartilage damage**

Inflammatory joint diseases like rheumatoid arthritis involve chronic inflammation of the joints, which can lead to progressive damage to the synovium (the lining of the joint) and surrounding tissues. The inflammation can affect the articular cartilage, leading to its breakdown and degeneration. Over time, the continuous inflammation and cartilage damage can contribute to the development of secondary osteoarthritis.

- **Altered joint mechanics**

Inflammatory joint diseases can also result in joint deformities, joint instability, and changes in joint mechanics. These alterations in joint structure and function can lead to uneven distribution of forces on the joint surfaces, increasing the wear and tear on specific areas of the cartilage. The altered mechanics can accelerate the degeneration process and increase the risk of developing secondary osteoarthritis.

- **Systemic inflammation**

Inflammatory joint diseases are characterized by systemic inflammation, meaning that the inflammation can affect the entire body. This systemic inflammation can contribute to the overall degeneration of joint tissues, including cartilage. The combination of local joint inflammation and systemic inflammation can further contribute to the development and progression of osteoarthritis in affected joints.

- **Treatment implications**

Managing inflammatory joint diseases like rheumatoid arthritis typically involves interventions to control inflammation, preserve joint function, and reduce symptoms. Adequate management of the underlying inflammatory condition is important in minimizing the risk of secondary osteoarthritis. Early diagnosis, appropriate medication, and other interventions to control inflammation can help slow down the progression of joint damage and potentially reduce the risk of secondary osteoarthritis.

- **Multidisciplinary approach**

Given the complex relationship between inflammatory joint diseases and secondary osteoarthritis, a multidisciplinary approach involving rheumatologists, orthopedic specialists, and other healthcare professionals is often necessary. This approach aims to address the underlying inflammatory condition, manage symptoms, and provide strategies to preserve joint function and minimize the impact of secondary osteoarthritis.

If you have an inflammatory joint disease such as rheumatoid arthritis, it is important to work closely with your healthcare team to manage your condition effectively. They can provide appropriate treatment options, lifestyle recommendations, and regular monitoring to help reduce the risk of secondary osteoarthritis and optimize your joint health.

16. Joint Infections

You are absolutely right. Joint infections, particularly septic arthritis, can have significant implications for joint health and increase the risk of developing osteoarthritis in the affected joint. Here are some key points regarding the relationship between joint infections and osteoarthritis:

- **Infection-induced joint damage**

Joint infections occur when bacteria or other infectious agents invade the joint space, leading to inflammation and damage to the joint structures. The infection can cause destruction of the articular cartilage, bone erosion, and disruption of the joint capsule and surrounding tissues. This damage can alter the joint mechanics and increase the risk of developing osteoarthritis.

- **Inflammatory response**

In response to the joint infection, the body's immune system activates an inflammatory response. While inflammation is a natural defense mechanism, prolonged or severe inflammation can lead to the breakdown of joint tissues, including cartilage. The persistent inflammation and tissue damage can contribute to the development of osteoarthritis in the affected joint.

- **Joint instability and altered mechanics**

Joint infections can result in joint instability and altered joint mechanics. The infection and associated tissue damage can lead to ligament laxity, joint deformities, and loss of normal joint alignment. These changes can result in uneven distribution of forces on the joint surfaces, increasing the risk of cartilage wear and tear and accelerating the development of osteoarthritis.

- **Delayed treatment or inadequate management**

Delayed diagnosis or inadequate treatment of joint infections can further increase the risk of complications, including the development of secondary osteoarthritis. Prompt identification and appropriate management of joint infections, including the use of antibiotics and drainage procedures if necessary, are crucial in minimizing joint damage and the subsequent risk of osteoarthritis.

- **Rehabilitation and follow-up care**

Following a joint infection, comprehensive rehabilitation and close follow-up care are essential. Rehabilitation aims to restore joint function, strength, and stability while minimizing the risk of complications. Regular follow-up appointments with healthcare providers can help monitor the joint's condition, identify any signs of osteoarthritis, and provide appropriate management strategies.

It's important to note that not all joint infections will lead to the development of osteoarthritis. Factors such as the severity and duration of the infection, prompt and effective treatment, and individual factors can influence the outcome. However, joint infections are considered a significant risk factor for subsequent osteoarthritis development in the affected joint.

If you have concerns about a joint infection or are experiencing joint symptoms after a previous infection, it is important to seek medical attention promptly. A healthcare professional can evaluate your condition, provide appropriate treatment, and offer guidance on rehabilitation and long-term joint health management to minimize the risk of osteoarthritis and promote optimal joint function.

17. Metabolic Disorders

Metabolic conditions such as diabetes and hemochromatosis have been associated with an increased risk of developing osteoarthritis. Here's a closer look at how these conditions can influence the development and progression of osteoarthritis:

1. Diabetes

Diabetes is a metabolic disorder characterized by high blood sugar levels. People with diabetes have an increased risk of developing osteoarthritis, particularly in weight-bearing joints such as the knees. Several factors contribute to this association:

- **Inflammation**

Diabetes is associated with chronic low-grade inflammation throughout the body. This inflammation can affect joint tissues, including cartilage, and contribute to its degeneration.

- **Insulin resistance**

Insulin resistance, a hallmark of type 2 diabetes, may lead to metabolic and hormonal imbalances that can negatively impact joint health. Insulin resistance can affect cartilage metabolism and increase the production of certain molecules that promote cartilage breakdown.

- **Obesity**

Diabetes is often associated with obesity, which is a known risk factor for osteoarthritis. Excess body weight places additional stress on the joints, accelerating cartilage degeneration.

- **Microvascular complications**

Diabetes can lead to microvascular complications, such as damage to small blood vessels. Impaired blood flow to the joints can limit the delivery of nutrients and oxygen, hindering the repair and maintenance of joint tissues.

2. Hemochromatosis

Hemochromatosis is a condition characterized by excessive iron accumulation in the body. Iron overload can affect joint health and increase the risk of osteoarthritis through several mechanisms:

- **Increased oxidative stress**

Excess iron can promote the generation of reactive oxygen species, leading to oxidative stress. This oxidative stress can damage joint tissues, including cartilage, and contribute to its degeneration.

- **Iron-induced inflammation**

Iron overload can trigger chronic low-grade inflammation in the body, which can affect joint tissues and promote the development of osteoarthritis.

- **Joint space narrowing**

Hemochromatosis can lead to joint space narrowing, a characteristic feature of osteoarthritis. The excessive iron deposition in joint tissues can disrupt their normal structure and function, leading to cartilage loss and joint degeneration.

It's important to note that while diabetes and hemochromatosis are associated with an increased risk of osteoarthritis, not all individuals with these conditions will develop osteoarthritis. Managing these metabolic conditions through appropriate medical care, lifestyle modifications, and regular monitoring can help reduce the risk and minimize the impact of osteoarthritis. Additionally, early detection and intervention for osteoarthritis symptoms are important for effective management and preserving joint function.

18. Genetic Predisposition

Genetic predisposition plays a significant role in the development of osteoarthritis. Here's a closer look at how genetics can influence the risk of osteoarthritis:

- **Genetic Variations**

Certain genetic variations or mutations can affect the structure, metabolism, and function of cartilage, making individuals more prone to developing osteoarthritis. These variations can impact the production and breakdown of collagen, proteoglycans, and other components of cartilage, leading to its degeneration.

- **Family History**

Having a family history of osteoarthritis can increase the risk of developing the condition. If one or both parents have osteoarthritis, their children are more likely to develop it as well. This suggests that genetic factors passed down through generations contribute to the susceptibility to osteoarthritis.

- **Gene Expression and Regulation**

Gene expression and regulation can be influenced by various factors, including environmental factors and lifestyle choices. Some studies suggest that environmental factors can interact with genetic factors, modulating gene expression and potentially affecting the risk of developing osteoarthritis.

It's important to note that while genetics plays a role in osteoarthritis, it is not the sole determinant. Other factors, such as age, joint stress, obesity, and previous joint injuries, also contribute to the development and progression of osteoarthritis. It is a complex interplay between genetic and environmental factors.

Understanding your genetic predisposition for osteoarthritis can provide valuable insights into your risk. However, it's essential to remember that having a genetic predisposition does not guarantee that you will develop osteoarthritis. Lifestyle choices, such as maintaining a healthy weight, engaging in regular physical activity, and protecting your joints from excessive stress, can help mitigate the risk and manage the condition effectively.

If you have a family history of osteoarthritis or suspect a genetic predisposition, it's advisable to consult with a healthcare professional or a genetic counselor. They can provide personalized guidance and help you make informed decisions about managing your risk and promoting joint health.

19. Joint Instability

Absolutely, joint instability is a significant risk factor for the development of osteoarthritis. Here's a closer look at how joint instability can contribute to the risk of osteoarthritis:

- **Structural Abnormalities**

Structural abnormalities in the joints, such as congenital abnormalities or previous joint injuries, can lead to joint instability. These abnormalities can affect the alignment, shape, or stability of the joint, resulting in uneven distribution of forces during movement. Over time, this imbalance places excessive stress on specific areas of the joint, leading to accelerated wear and tear of the cartilage.

- **Joint Laxity**

Joint laxity refers to excessive joint looseness or hypermobility. Some individuals naturally have more lax joints due to genetic factors or connective tissue disorders. Joint laxity can affect the stability and support of the joint, making it more vulnerable to injury and cartilage damage. Chronic instability due to joint laxity can contribute to the development of osteoarthritis.

- **Ligament or Capsule Tears**

Injuries to the ligaments or joint capsule, such as ligament tears or sprains, can result in joint instability. When the supporting structures of the joint are damaged, they are unable to provide adequate stability, leading to increased stress on the joint surfaces. This can accelerate cartilage degeneration and increase the risk of osteoarthritis.

It's important to address joint instability to reduce the risk of osteoarthritis. Treatment options for joint instability may include physical therapy to strengthen the muscles surrounding the joint, bracing or orthotic devices to provide additional support, or, in severe cases, surgical interventions to repair or reconstruct the damaged structures.

If you have joint instability or suspect that your joints are unstable, it's crucial to consult with a healthcare professional or an orthopedic specialist. They can assess your joint stability, provide appropriate treatment recommendations, and guide you on strategies to protect your joints and minimize the risk of osteoarthritis.

20. Poor Joint Alignment

Absolutely, poor joint alignment is a significant factor that can contribute to the development of osteoarthritis. When joints are not properly aligned, it can lead to uneven distribution of forces during movement, resulting in increased stress on certain areas of the joint. Over time, this can lead to accelerated wear and tear of the cartilage, cartilage degradation, and the development of osteoarthritis. Here are a few examples of how poor joint alignment can affect different joints:

- **Bowed Legs**

Bowed legs, also known as genu varum, is a condition where the legs curve outward, causing the knees to be farther apart than the ankles when standing. This alignment issue can place excessive stress on the inner side of the knee joint. The increased pressure on the inner compartment of the knee can lead to cartilage damage and the development of osteoarthritis in that area.

- **Unequal Leg Length**

Having a significant difference in leg length, known as leg length discrepancy, can result in abnormal forces on the joints. The uneven weight distribution can affect the alignment and stability of the joints, particularly in the hips, knees, and ankles. Over time, this imbalance can contribute to cartilage breakdown and increase the risk of osteoarthritis.

- **Patellar Tracking Issues**

Patellar tracking refers to the movement of the kneecap (patella) during knee flexion and extension. If the patella does not track properly within the groove of the femur, it can cause abnormal stress on the cartilage surface behind the patella. This can lead to cartilage damage, pain, and the development of osteoarthritis in the patellofemoral joint.

Addressing poor joint alignment is essential to reduce the risk of osteoarthritis. Treatment options may include physical therapy to correct muscle imbalances and improve joint stability, orthotic devices or braces to support proper alignment, or in some cases, surgical interventions to realign the joint structures.

If you have concerns about poor joint alignment or notice any abnormalities in your joints, it's important to consult with a healthcare professional or an orthopedic specialist. They can evaluate your joint alignment, provide appropriate interventions or recommendations, and help you prevent or manage osteoarthritis associated with poor joint alignment.

It is important to note that the presence of these risk factors does not guarantee the development of osteoarthritis. Osteoarthritis is a complex condition influenced by a combination of factors, and each individual's experience with the disease may vary. By understanding the potential causes and risk factors, individuals can take proactive measures to reduce their risk and manage the condition effectively.

The Impact of Osteoarthritis on Daily Life

Osteoarthritis can have a significant impact on daily life, affecting various aspects of physical, emotional, and social well-being. Here are some ways in which osteoarthritis can impact daily life:

1. Pain and Discomfort

Osteoarthritis often causes joint pain, stiffness, and swelling, which can vary in intensity. The pain may worsen with movement or weight-bearing activities, making it challenging to perform daily tasks and activities that require joint mobility. Simple actions like walking, climbing stairs, or getting up from a chair can become difficult and painful.

2. Reduced Mobility and Function

As osteoarthritis progresses, it can lead to a gradual loss of joint function and mobility. Joint stiffness, limited range of motion, and muscle weakness can make it harder to perform activities that were once routine. This may include difficulty with dressing, bathing, cooking, and other self-care tasks.

3. Impact on Physical Activity

Osteoarthritis can significantly affect physical activity levels. The fear of pain or worsening joint damage may lead individuals to avoid exercise and reduce their overall physical activity. This can have a negative impact on cardiovascular health, muscle strength, and overall fitness.

4. Emotional Well-being

Chronic pain and limitations in daily activities can take a toll on emotional well-being. Osteoarthritis can cause frustration, sadness, stress, and anxiety. Coping with the physical and emotional challenges of osteoarthritis may require significant adjustment and support.

5. Sleep Disturbances

Pain and discomfort from osteoarthritis can interfere with sleep quality and duration. Joint pain may worsen at night, making it difficult to find a comfortable sleeping position. Sleep disturbances can further contribute to fatigue and impact overall well-being.

6. Impact on Work and Productivity

Osteoarthritis can affect work performance and productivity. Joint pain, reduced mobility, and limitations in physical activity can make it challenging to carry out job responsibilities, particularly for those with physically demanding occupations.

7. Social Impact

Osteoarthritis can affect social interactions and participation in social activities. Individuals may experience difficulties attending social events, participating in hobbies, or engaging in recreational activities due to pain and physical limitations. This can lead to feelings of isolation, withdrawal, and decreased quality of life.

8. Limitations in Daily Activities

Osteoarthritis can impact daily activities that were once taken for granted. Simple tasks like cooking, cleaning, shopping, and running errands may become challenging or require modifications to accommodate joint pain and limitations. This can lead to a loss of independence and reliance on others for assistance.

9. Emotional Impact

Osteoarthritis can have a profound emotional impact on individuals. Chronic pain, limitations in daily activities, and the potential for long-term disability can lead to feelings of frustration, sadness, and helplessness. Coping with the emotional aspects of osteoarthritis, such as adjusting to a new lifestyle and managing expectations, is crucial for overall well-being.

10. Reduced Quality of Life

The cumulative impact of pain, physical limitations, and emotional distress can significantly reduce an individual's quality of life. Osteoarthritis may restrict participation in enjoyable activities, hobbies, and social events, leading to a diminished sense of fulfillment and satisfaction.

11. Financial Burden

Osteoarthritis can impose a financial burden on individuals and their families. The cost of medical treatments, medications, assistive devices, and modifications to living spaces can add up over time. Additionally, reduced work productivity or the inability to work due to osteoarthritis-related limitations may result in financial strain.

12. Caregiver Burden

Osteoarthritis not only affects the individuals living with the condition but also places a burden on their caregivers. Family members or friends providing assistance and support may experience physical and emotional strain, as they often take on additional responsibilities and witness the challenges faced by their loved ones.

It is important for individuals with osteoarthritis to seek appropriate medical care, develop a comprehensive management plan, and engage in self-care practices. This may involve a combination of pain management strategies, exercise programs, physical therapy, assistive devices, and emotional support. By effectively managing the impact of osteoarthritis, individuals can improve their overall well-being and maintain a fulfilling and active lifestyle to the best of their abilities.

Chapter 2

Types of Osteoarthritis

Osteoarthritis can be classified into different types based on the specific joints affected. These types encompass the major areas where osteoarthritis commonly occurs. It's important to note that while these are the primary types, osteoarthritis can also affect other joints in the body, albeit less frequently. The classification of osteoarthritis helps in understanding the location and specific characteristics of the condition, allowing for targeted treatment approaches and management strategies.

Here are some common types of osteoarthritis:

1. Knee Osteoarthritis

Knee osteoarthritis is the most prevalent form of osteoarthritis and affects the knee joints. It occurs when the protective cartilage that cushions the ends of the bones in the knee joint gradually wears and tears away over time. This can lead to pain, stiffness, swelling, and difficulty in movement. The risk factors for knee osteoarthritis include age, obesity, previous knee injuries, repetitive stress on the joint, genetics, and certain occupations that involve kneeling or heavy lifting.

Treatment for knee osteoarthritis focuses on managing symptoms and improving joint function. It may involve a combination of lifestyle changes, such as weight loss and exercise, pain management with medications or injections, physical therapy, assistive devices like braces or canes, and in severe cases, surgical interventions like arthroscopy or knee replacement. Proper diagnosis and individualized treatment plans are essential for managing knee osteoarthritis effectively.

2. Hip Osteoarthritis

Hip osteoarthritis is a common form of osteoarthritis that affects the hip joints. It occurs when the cartilage that covers the ends of the bones in the hip joint wears down, leading to pain, stiffness, and reduced range of motion.

The exact cause of hip osteoarthritis is often a combination of factors, including age, genetics, joint injury, obesity, and repetitive stress on the joint. Symptoms of hip osteoarthritis can include hip pain, which may radiate to the groin, thigh, or buttocks, stiffness, difficulty in walking or performing activities like getting up from a seated position or climbing stairs, and a decrease in hip joint mobility.

Treatment options for hip osteoarthritis include lifestyle modifications such as weight management and low-impact exercise, pain relief medications, physical therapy, assistive devices like canes or walkers, and in severe cases, surgical interventions such as hip replacement surgery. Proper diagnosis and a comprehensive treatment plan tailored to the individual's needs can help manage hip osteoarthritis and improve quality of life.

3. Hand Osteoarthritis

Hand osteoarthritis is a type of osteoarthritis that primarily affects the joints of the fingers, thumb, and wrist. It is characterized by the gradual breakdown of the cartilage in these joints, leading to pain, stiffness, and reduced function. Hand osteoarthritis can occur due to a combination of factors, including aging, genetics, previous joint injuries, and repetitive hand movements or occupations that involve manual labor.

Symptoms of hand osteoarthritis may include joint pain, swelling, stiffness, tenderness, and the development of bony nodules called

Heberden's nodes or Bouchard's nodes. These nodes can be visible or felt as small, hard bumps near the joints. Treatment for hand osteoarthritis focuses on managing symptoms and improving hand function.

It may include lifestyle modifications, such as protecting the hands during activities and using assistive devices for support, pain relief medications, topical treatments, splints or braces to support the joints, hand exercises or physical therapy, and, in severe cases, surgery to repair or replace damaged joints. An accurate diagnosis and a personalized treatment plan can help individuals with hand osteoarthritis manage their symptoms and maintain hand function.

4. Spine Osteoarthritis

Spine osteoarthritis, also known as spinal osteoarthritis or degenerative disc disease, refers to the degeneration of the joints and discs in the spine. It commonly affects the neck (cervical spine) and lower back (lumbar spine). Spinal osteoarthritis is primarily a result of age-related wear and tear on the spine, but it can also be influenced by factors such as genetics, previous injuries, and certain lifestyle factors.

The symptoms of spine osteoarthritis can vary but often include pain, stiffness, and reduced flexibility in the affected region of the spine. The pain may be localized to the neck or lower back or can radiate to the arms, legs, or buttocks, depending on the location and severity of the condition. Other symptoms may include muscle weakness, numbness or tingling sensations, and difficulty with balance or coordination.

Treatment for spine osteoarthritis focuses on managing symptoms and improving the individual's quality of life. This can involve a combination of conservative measures, including pain medications, physical therapy, exercises to improve strength and flexibility, heat or cold therapy, and lifestyle modifications such as maintaining a healthy weight and avoiding activities that worsen symptoms.

In some cases, more advanced interventions may be considered, such as injections of corticosteroids or local anesthetics, spinal manipulation or mobilization, and in severe cases, surgery may be recommended to stabilize or decompress the affected area of the spine.

It's important to note that spine osteoarthritis is a chronic condition that requires ongoing management and a multidisciplinary approach involving healthcare professionals such as physicians, physical therapists, and pain specialists. The treatment plan is tailored to each individual's specific needs and aims to alleviate pain, improve function, and enhance overall well-being.

5. Shoulder Osteoarthritis

Shoulder osteoarthritis, also known as glenohumeral osteoarthritis, is a condition characterized by the degeneration of the cartilage in the shoulder joint. It typically occurs as a result of wear and tear over time, previous shoulder injuries, or conditions that affect the joint mechanics.

The primary symptoms of shoulder osteoarthritis include shoulder pain, stiffness, and reduced range of motion. Individuals may experience pain that worsens with movement or activities that require the use of the shoulder joint, such as reaching or lifting. Stiffness in the shoulder joint can make it challenging to perform daily tasks and may lead to a decreased range of motion.

Treatment for shoulder osteoarthritis aims to alleviate pain, improve function, and enhance the individual's quality of life. Conservative treatment options are often the initial approach and can include pain management with over-the-counter pain relievers, such as nonsteroidal anti-inflammatory drugs (NSAIDs), to reduce pain and inflammation. In some cases, corticosteroid injections into the shoulder joint can provide short-term pain relief.

Physical therapy is an important component of treatment for shoulder osteoarthritis. A physical therapist can prescribe specific exercises and stretches to improve shoulder strength, flexibility, and range of motion. They may also incorporate modalities such as heat or cold therapy, ultrasound, or electrical stimulation to help reduce pain and enhance healing.

In addition to medication and physical therapy, assistive devices like slings, braces, or orthotics can provide support, stability, and relief of stress on the shoulder joint. Lifestyle modifications are also important, including avoiding activities that aggravate symptoms and incorporating proper ergonomics and body mechanics to reduce strain on the shoulder joint.

In cases where conservative treatments are ineffective or if there is significant joint damage, surgical interventions may be considered. These can range from minimally invasive procedures like arthroscopy to repair or clean the joint, to more extensive surgeries like joint resurfacing or shoulder replacement.

It's essential for individuals with shoulder osteoarthritis to work closely with healthcare professionals, such as orthopedic specialists or physical therapists, to develop an individualized treatment plan that addresses their specific needs and goals. Regular follow-up appointments and adherence to the prescribed treatment plan can help manage symptoms, improve shoulder function, and enhance overall quality of life.

6. Foot and Ankle Osteoarthritis

Foot and ankle osteoarthritis is a condition characterized by the degeneration of the joints in the feet and ankles, leading to pain, swelling, stiffness, and difficulty in walking. It can be caused by factors such as previous injuries, repetitive stress on the joints, or structural abnormalities.

The treatment for foot and ankle osteoarthritis focuses on managing symptoms, reducing pain, and improving mobility. Conservative measures often include wearing supportive and cushioned footwear, using orthotic inserts or shoe modifications, and engaging in physical therapy to strengthen the muscles around the affected joints and improve range of motion. Pain relief medications, such as over-the-counter NSAIDs, may be recommended to alleviate pain and reduce inflammation. In more severe cases, corticosteroid injections into the affected joints or surgical interventions like joint fusion or replacement may be considered.

Individuals with foot and ankle osteoarthritis should seek medical advice from a healthcare professional, such as a podiatrist or orthopedic specialist, for an accurate diagnosis and to develop a personalized treatment plan. Adhering to the prescribed treatment, making lifestyle modifications, and maintaining regular follow-up appointments can help manage symptoms, slow down the progression of the condition, and improve overall foot and ankle function.

It's important to note that these types of osteoarthritis can often coexist or affect multiple joints simultaneously. The specific symptoms and management approaches may vary depending on the type and severity of osteoarthritis present. A healthcare professional can provide a comprehensive evaluation and appropriate treatment options tailored to individual needs.

Chapter 3

Diagnosing Osteoarthritis

Diagnosing osteoarthritis involves a thorough evaluation of the patient's symptoms, medical history, and physical examination findings. Imaging tests like X-rays and MRI scans help visualize joint damage and rule out other conditions, while joint fluid analysis and blood tests may be used to exclude alternative causes of symptoms. However, the diagnosis of osteoarthritis primarily relies on the patient's reported symptoms, clinical assessment of joint pain, stiffness, and limited mobility, along with characteristic signs observed during physical examination. An accurate diagnosis is crucial for developing an appropriate treatment plan and managing osteoarthritis effectively.

Recognizing the Symptoms

Recognizing the symptoms of osteoarthritis is crucial for early detection and appropriate management of the condition. Here are some common signs and symptoms to look out for:

1. Joint pain

Osteoarthritis typically presents with pain in the affected joints. The pain may be described as a dull ache or a sharp sensation and is often worse with movement or weight-bearing activities.

2. Joint stiffness

Stiffness in the joints, especially after periods of inactivity or upon waking up in the morning, is a common symptom of osteoarthritis. It may take some time for the joints to loosen up and regain their full range of motion.

3. Joint swelling

Inflammation and swelling can occur in the affected joints. The swelling is usually localized and may be accompanied by warmth and tenderness.

4. Joint instability

Osteoarthritis can lead to joint instability, making the affected joint feel loose or wobbly. This instability can affect mobility and increase the risk of falls or injuries.

5. Reduced range of motion

Over time, osteoarthritis can cause a decrease in joint flexibility and range of motion. This can make it challenging to perform everyday activities that require joint movement.

6. Joint deformities

In advanced cases, osteoarthritis can result in joint deformities, such as the formation of bony growths or nodes around the affected joints.

7. Grating or clicking sensation

Some individuals with osteoarthritis may experience a grating or clicking sensation when moving the affected joint. This can be due to the roughening of the joint surfaces or the presence of loose fragments within the joint.

8. Muscle weakness

Osteoarthritis can lead to muscle weakness around the affected joint. This weakness may occur as a result of pain or reduced usage of the joint, leading to muscle atrophy and decreased strength.

9. Limited function and difficulty performing daily activities

As osteoarthritis progresses, individuals may find it increasingly challenging to perform daily activities that involve the affected joint, such as walking, climbing stairs, or gripping objects.

10. Fatigue

Ongoing pain and limited mobility associated with osteoarthritis can cause fatigue and exhaustion, particularly after engaging in activities that strain the affected joint.

It's important to remember that the symptoms of osteoarthritis can vary in severity and progression among individuals. If you experience any of these symptoms persistently or if they significantly impact your quality of life, it is recommended to consult a healthcare professional for an accurate diagnosis and appropriate management. They can conduct a physical examination, review your medical history, and order imaging tests, such as X-rays or MRIs, to confirm the presence of osteoarthritis and develop a tailored treatment plan. Early diagnosis and intervention can help slow down the progression of the disease, manage symptoms effectively, and improve overall joint function.

Diagnostic Tests and Imaging Techniques

Diagnostic tests and imaging techniques play a crucial role in the diagnosis and evaluation of osteoarthritis. Here are some commonly used methods:

1. X-rays

X-rays are the most common imaging technique used to diagnose osteoarthritis. They can help visualize the joint space, identify joint damage, and detect the presence of bone spurs or osteophytes. X-rays can also determine the degree of joint degeneration and aid in monitoring disease progression.

2. Magnetic Resonance Imaging (MRI)

MRI scans provide detailed images of the soft tissues, cartilage, and bones. They can help assess the extent of joint damage, identify areas of inflammation, and evaluate the condition of the surrounding structures. MRI scans are particularly useful when evaluating joints with complex anatomy or when further characterization of the joint is required.

3. Computed Tomography (CT) scan

CT scans use a series of X-ray images to create cross-sectional images of the joint. They can provide detailed views of the bones, joints, and surrounding structures. CT scans are useful in evaluating complex joint deformities or when more precise information about the joint is needed.

4. Ultrasound

Ultrasound uses sound waves to create real-time images of the joint structures. It can help visualize joint inflammation, assess the thickness of the joint lining (synovium), and identify the presence of fluid accumulation or cysts. Ultrasound is often used for guided joint injections or to assess joint effusion.

5. Joint aspiration

Joint aspiration, also known as arthrocentesis, involves the removal of fluid from the affected joint. The collected fluid is then analyzed for signs of inflammation, infection, or other conditions that may mimic osteoarthritis.

6. Blood tests

While there is no specific blood test to diagnose osteoarthritis, blood tests can be helpful in ruling out other conditions that may have similar symptoms. Blood tests can help identify markers of inflammation and rule out other forms of arthritis, such as rheumatoid arthritis or gout.

7. Bone scans

Bone scans involve the injection of a radioactive substance into the bloodstream, which is then taken up by the bones. The scan detects areas of increased bone metabolism, which can indicate joint inflammation or degeneration. Bone scans are typically used when other imaging techniques are inconclusive or when multiple joints are affected.

8. Physical examination

A thorough physical examination by a healthcare professional can provide valuable information about joint tenderness, swelling, range of motion, and overall joint function. The physical examination, combined with the patient's medical history and symptoms, can aid in the diagnosis of osteoarthritis.

It's important to note that no single test can definitively diagnose osteoarthritis. Instead, a combination of clinical evaluation, imaging studies, and other tests are used to make an accurate diagnosis. The choice of diagnostic tests depends on various factors, including the specific joint affected, the severity of symptoms, and the clinical judgment of the healthcare professional.

While imaging techniques are valuable in diagnosing osteoarthritis, it is important to note that clinical evaluation and patient history are equally important. A healthcare professional will consider a combination of symptoms, physical examination findings, and imaging results to make an accurate diagnosis and develop an appropriate treatment plan.

Consulting with Healthcare Professionals

Consulting with healthcare professionals is essential for the diagnosis, treatment, and management of osteoarthritis. Here's why it's important to seek medical advice:

1. Accurate diagnosis

Healthcare professionals, such as primary care physicians or rheumatologists, have the expertise to properly diagnose osteoarthritis. They will assess your symptoms, conduct a physical examination, review your medical history, and order appropriate tests or imaging studies to confirm the diagnosis. Getting an accurate diagnosis is crucial for developing an effective treatment plan.

2. Tailored treatment plan

Healthcare professionals will develop a personalized treatment plan based on your specific needs and the severity of your osteoarthritis. They may recommend a combination of treatments, such as medications to manage pain and inflammation, physical therapy exercises to improve joint function and mobility, assistive devices to support joints, and lifestyle modifications to reduce stress on the joints.

3. Monitoring disease progression

Regular follow-up visits with healthcare professionals allow them to monitor the progression of osteoarthritis and make any necessary adjustments to the treatment plan. They can track changes in symptoms, assess joint function, and determine if additional interventions or therapies are needed.

4. Education and guidance

Healthcare professionals can provide valuable education and guidance about osteoarthritis. They can explain the nature of the condition, discuss risk factors, provide advice on lifestyle modifications (e.g., weight management, exercise, joint protection), and offer strategies for pain management and self-care.

5. Referrals to specialists

In some cases, healthcare professionals may refer you to specialists, such as orthopedic surgeons or physical therapists, for further evaluation or specialized care. Specialists can offer expertise in specific areas, such as joint surgery or advanced rehabilitation techniques, to optimize your treatment outcomes.

Remember, healthcare professionals have the knowledge and experience to provide appropriate guidance and support for managing osteoarthritis. Regular communication and collaboration with them are key to effectively managing your condition and improving your quality of life.

Chapter 4

Managing Osteoarthritis Pain

Managing osteoarthritis involves a comprehensive approach that includes pain management, exercise, and weight management. The primary goal is to reduce pain, improve joint function, and enhance overall quality of life. Pain management strategies may involve the use of medications, both over-the-counter and prescription, to alleviate pain and inflammation.

Topical treatments can also be applied directly to the affected joints for localized relief. In addition to medication, regular exercise is crucial for strengthening the muscles around the joints, improving joint flexibility, and maintaining overall joint health. Low-impact activities like walking, swimming, and cycling are often recommended to minimize joint stress.

Weight management is another important aspect of osteoarthritis management, as excess weight places additional stress on the joints. Maintaining a healthy weight or achieving weight loss can reduce the burden on the joints, leading to decreased pain and improved mobility.

Consulting with healthcare professionals, such as physicians and physical therapists, is essential for developing an individualized management plan that addresses your specific needs and goals. They can provide guidance on medication use, prescribe appropriate exercises, and offer support throughout your journey of managing osteoarthritis.

Over-the-Counter Pain Relief Options

Over-the-counter (OTC) pain relief options can be effective in managing mild to moderate pain associated with osteoarthritis. Here are some common OTC pain relief options:

1. Acetaminophen (Tylenol)

Acetaminophen is a commonly used pain reliever that can help reduce osteoarthritis pain. It is generally considered safe and can be effective for mild to moderate pain. However, it's important to follow the recommended dosage and avoid exceeding the maximum daily limit to prevent potential liver damage.

2. Nonsteroidal Anti-Inflammatory Drugs (NSAIDs)

NSAIDs, such as ibuprofen (Advil, Motrin) and naproxen (Aleve), are OTC medications that can help reduce pain and inflammation associated with osteoarthritis. They work by reducing the production of certain chemicals in the body that contribute to pain and swelling. It's important to use NSAIDs as directed and be aware of potential side effects, such as stomach upset or increased risk of bleeding.

3. Topical Analgesics

Topical analgesics are creams, gels, or patches that can be applied directly to the affected joints to provide localized pain relief. They often contain ingredients like menthol, camphor, or salicylates that help alleviate pain. These products can be a good option for individuals who prefer to avoid oral medications or have localized pain in specific joints.

It's important to consult with a healthcare professional or pharmacist before using OTC pain relief options to ensure they are safe and appropriate for your specific situation. They can provide guidance on proper usage, potential interactions with other medications, and help determine the most suitable option for managing your osteoarthritis pain.

Prescription Medications for Pain Management

Prescription medications can be prescribed by healthcare professionals to manage moderate to severe pain associated with osteoarthritis. Here are some common prescription medications used for pain management:

1. Nonsteroidal Anti-Inflammatory Drugs (NSAIDs)

Prescription-strength NSAIDs, such as celecoxib (Celebrex), diclofenac (Voltaren), or meloxicam (Mobic), may be prescribed to manage pain and inflammation in osteoarthritis. These medications are more potent than their over-the-counter counterparts and may provide greater pain relief. However, they carry a higher risk of side effects, particularly gastrointestinal issues and cardiovascular risks. Close monitoring by a healthcare professional is important when using prescription-strength NSAIDs.

2. Opioids

In some cases, opioids may be prescribed for severe osteoarthritis pain that does not respond to other medications. Medications like oxycodone (OxyContin), tramadol (Ultram), or codeine may be used. Opioids can effectively relieve pain but come with risks, including dependence, addiction, and side effects such as constipation and drowsiness. Due to these risks, opioids are typically used cautiously and for a limited duration.

3. Duloxetine

Duloxetine (Cymbalta) is an antidepressant that is also approved for treating chronic pain, including osteoarthritis. It works by increasing the levels of certain neurotransmitters in the brain that help regulate pain perception. Duloxetine may be prescribed to manage both pain and associated symptoms of depression or anxiety.

4. Topical Analgesics

Prescription-strength topical analgesics, such as lidocaine patches or compounded creams, may be prescribed for localized pain relief. These formulations can be applied directly to the affected joints to numb the area and provide temporary pain relief.

It's important to note that prescription medications should be used under the guidance of a healthcare professional. They will assess your condition, consider your medical history, and tailor the prescription to your specific needs. Regular follow-ups are essential to monitor the effectiveness of the medication and address any potential side effects or concerns.

Exploring Non-Pharmacological Pain Relief Techniques

In addition to medication, there are various non-pharmacological techniques that can help provide pain relief and improve the management of osteoarthritis. These techniques focus on reducing pain, improving joint function, and enhancing overall well-being.

Here are some commonly used non-pharmacological pain relief techniques:

1. Physical therapy

Physical therapy plays a crucial role in managing osteoarthritis pain. A physical therapist can develop an individualized exercise program that includes specific exercises to strengthen the muscles around the affected joints, improve joint flexibility, and enhance overall joint function. They may also incorporate other techniques such as manual therapy, joint mobilization, and modalities like heat or cold therapy.

2. Occupational therapy

Occupational therapy focuses on improving the ability to perform daily activities while minimizing joint strain. An occupational therapist can provide guidance on joint protection techniques, assistive devices, and modifications to your home or workplace to make activities easier and reduce pain.

3. Weight management

Maintaining a healthy weight or achieving weight loss, if necessary, can significantly reduce the burden on the joints and alleviate pain. Excess weight places additional stress on the joints, particularly weight-bearing joints like the knees and hips. Working with a healthcare professional or a registered dietitian can help develop a personalized weight management plan.

4. Assistive devices

The use of assistive devices can help reduce joint stress and improve mobility. Examples include using canes or walking aids to offload weight from the affected joints, wearing supportive shoes or orthotics to provide cushioning and stability, or using braces or splints to provide joint support.

5. Heat and cold therapy

Applying heat or cold to the affected joints can help relieve pain and reduce inflammation. Heat therapy, such as warm baths, hot packs, or heating pads, can help relax muscles and improve circulation. Cold therapy, such as ice packs or cold compresses, can numb the area and reduce swelling.

6. Transcutaneous Electrical Nerve Stimulation (TENS)

TENS is a technique that uses low-voltage electrical currents to stimulate nerves and provide pain relief. It involves placing electrodes on the skin near the affected joint to deliver gentle electrical impulses, which can help disrupt pain signals and promote the release of endorphins.

7. Mind-body techniques

Techniques like meditation, deep breathing exercises, and relaxation techniques can help manage pain by reducing stress, promoting relaxation, and improving overall well-being. These techniques can be particularly helpful in managing the emotional and psychological aspects of living with chronic pain.

8. Acupuncture

Acupuncture is an ancient Chinese practice that involves inserting thin needles into specific points on the body. It is believed to help restore the balance of energy, known as Qi, and promote pain relief. Acupuncture has been found to be effective in reducing pain and improving joint function in individuals with osteoarthritis.

9. Hydrotherapy

Hydrotherapy, also known as aquatic therapy, involves performing exercises in a warm water pool. The buoyancy of the water reduces stress on the joints while providing resistance for strengthening. Hydrotherapy can improve joint mobility, reduce pain, and enhance overall physical function.

10. Cognitive-behavioral therapy (CBT)

CBT is a therapeutic approach that focuses on changing negative thoughts, beliefs, and behaviors related to pain. It can help individuals with osteoarthritis develop coping strategies, manage stress, and improve their overall quality of life.

11. Dietary modifications

Certain dietary changes may help reduce inflammation and improve symptoms of osteoarthritis. A diet rich in anti-inflammatory foods, such as fruits, vegetables, whole grains, and fatty fish, can have a positive impact on joint health. Additionally, avoiding or reducing the consumption of processed foods, sugary drinks, and foods high in saturated and trans fats may help manage symptoms.

It's important to consult with healthcare professionals or specialists in these areas to determine the most suitable non-pharmacological techniques for your specific needs and to receive proper guidance on their implementation. Integrating a combination of these techniques into your daily routine can help improve pain management and overall quality of life.

Chapter 5

Lifestyle Modifications for Osteoarthritis

Osteoarthritis is a chronic condition characterized by the degeneration of joint cartilage and the underlying bone. While there is no cure for osteoarthritis, lifestyle modifications can help manage symptoms, reduce pain, and improve overall quality of life. Here are some lifestyle modifications that may be beneficial for individuals with osteoarthritis:

1. **Exercise regularly**

Low-impact exercises such as walking, swimming, cycling, and tai chi can help strengthen muscles around the joints, improve flexibility, and reduce pain. Consult with a healthcare professional or a physical therapist to develop a personalized exercise program.

2. **Maintain a healthy weight**

Excess weight places additional stress on weight-bearing joints, such as the knees and hips. Losing weight, if necessary, can significantly reduce the load on these joints and alleviate symptoms.

3. **Protect your joints**

Avoid activities that place excessive strain on your joints, such as high-impact sports or activities that involve repetitive joint movements. Use joint supports or assistive devices (e.g., braces, canes, or splints) when needed to provide extra support and reduce joint stress.

4. Practice good posture

Maintaining proper posture can help distribute the load on your joints more evenly. When sitting, choose an ergonomic chair with good back support, and avoid slouching. When standing, distribute your weight evenly on both feet.

5. Modify your activities

Make adjustments to your daily activities to reduce joint stress. For example, use proper lifting techniques, avoid prolonged kneeling or squatting, and take frequent breaks if you engage in activities that require repetitive motions.

6. Apply heat or cold therapy

Applying heat or cold to affected joints can help alleviate pain and reduce inflammation. Heat therapy, such as warm showers or heating pads, can help relax muscles and improve blood circulation. Cold therapy, such as ice packs or cold compresses, can help reduce swelling and numb pain.

7. Consider physical therapy

A physical therapist can provide targeted exercises and treatments to help manage osteoarthritis symptoms. They can guide you on proper movement techniques, joint protection strategies, and assistive devices that may be beneficial.

8. Eat a balanced diet

Consuming a healthy, well-balanced diet rich in fruits, vegetables, whole grains, lean proteins, and healthy fats can support overall joint health. Certain foods, such as fatty fish (e.g., salmon), nuts, and seeds, may have anti-inflammatory properties. Additionally, maintaining adequate hydration is important for joint lubrication.

9. Get sufficient rest and sleep

Rest and sleep are essential for joint healing and overall well-being. Ensure you have a comfortable mattress and pillow that provide adequate support. If necessary, use pillows or cushions to support joints while sleeping.

10. Manage stress

Chronic pain from osteoarthritis can take a toll on mental health. Engage in stress-reducing activities such as meditation, deep breathing exercises, yoga, or hobbies that help you relax and unwind.

11. Use assistive devices

Assistive devices, such as shoe orthotics, splints, or canes, can help relieve pressure on joints and improve mobility. Talk to your healthcare professional about appropriate assistive devices for your specific needs.

12. Avoid prolonged inactivity

While rest is important, prolonged inactivity can lead to joint stiffness and muscle weakness. Engage in regular, low-impact activities to keep joints mobile and muscles strong.

13. Balance rest and activity

Find the right balance between rest and activity. Listen to your body and pace yourself to avoid overexertion. Take breaks when needed, but try to stay active to maintain joint flexibility.

14. Quit smoking

Smoking has been linked to increased inflammation and cartilage damage. If you smoke, quitting can help improve your overall joint health and reduce osteoarthritis symptoms.

15. Manage pain

Use pain management techniques, such as over-the-counter pain relievers, topical creams, or prescription medications as recommended by your healthcare professional. Physical therapy techniques like massage, transcutaneous electrical nerve stimulation (TENS), or acupuncture may also provide pain relief.

16. Stay educated

Learn about osteoarthritis, its management, and treatment options. Stay up-to-date with current research and advancements in the field. Being informed can empower you to make better decisions regarding your condition.

17. Consider complementary therapies

Some individuals find relief from osteoarthritis symptoms through complementary therapies such as acupuncture, herbal supplements, or mind-body techniques like meditation or yoga. Consult with your healthcare professional before trying any complementary therapies to ensure they are safe and appropriate for you.

It's important to consult with a healthcare professional for personalized advice and recommendations based on your specific condition and needs. They can provide guidance tailored to your situation and may suggest additional treatments or interventions to manage osteoarthritis effectively.

Importance of Exercise and Physical Activity

Exercise and physical activity play a crucial role in maintaining overall health and well-being. Here are some key reasons why exercise and physical activity are important:

1. Physical health

Regular exercise and physical activity have numerous benefits for physical health. They help maintain a healthy weight, improve cardiovascular health, strengthen muscles and bones, enhance flexibility and balance, and reduce the risk of chronic conditions such as heart disease, diabetes, and certain types of cancer.

2. Mental health

Exercise has a positive impact on mental health and can help reduce symptoms of stress, anxiety, and depression. It promotes the release of endorphins, which are natural mood-enhancing chemicals in the brain. Regular physical activity can boost self-esteem, improve sleep patterns, and enhance cognitive function.

3. Weight management

Engaging in regular exercise and physical activity is an effective way to manage weight. It helps burn calories and build muscle mass, which increases metabolism. By maintaining a healthy weight, individuals reduce the risk of obesity-related conditions and improve overall health.

4. Disease prevention

Exercise and physical activity contribute to the prevention of various chronic diseases. Regular physical activity reduces the risk of cardiovascular diseases, such as heart disease and stroke. It also helps lower the risk of developing type 2 diabetes, certain types of cancer (such as colon and breast cancer), and osteoporosis.

5. Improved quality of life

Regular exercise and physical activity enhance overall quality of life. They improve energy levels, increase stamina, and enhance the ability to perform daily tasks and activities. Exercise can also improve mobility, flexibility, and balance, reducing the risk of falls and injuries.

6. Social interaction

Participating in group exercises or team sports can provide opportunities for social interaction and community engagement. This can contribute to a sense of belonging, camaraderie, and overall social well-being.

7. Cognitive function

Exercise has been shown to have a positive impact on cognitive function and brain health. It improves memory, attention, and executive functions. Regular physical activity may also reduce the risk of cognitive decline and improve overall brain health, particularly in older adults.

It's important to note that individuals should consult with a healthcare professional before starting any new exercise program, especially if they have underlying health conditions or concerns. They can provide personalized recommendations based on individual needs and abilities.

Weight Management Strategies

Weight management strategies refer to the practices and techniques used to achieve and maintain a healthy body weight. These strategies typically involve a combination of healthy eating habits, regular physical activity, behavior modification, and lifestyle changes. The goal is to achieve a balance between energy intake (calories consumed) and energy expenditure (calories burned) in order to reach and maintain a healthy weight.

Weight management is important for overall health, as it can reduce the risk of chronic diseases, improve physical fitness, and enhance well-being.

Here are some strategies for effective weight management:

1. Set realistic goals

Setting realistic goals is essential for effective weight management. It's important to be specific about what you want to achieve, whether it's losing a certain amount of weight or fitting into a particular clothing size. Avoid vague goals and instead focus on clear and measurable targets that you can work towards.

Achievability is key when setting weight management goals. Consider your current lifestyle, commitments, and health status. Setting goals that are within reach increases your chances of success and keeps you motivated. Avoid setting unrealistic expectations that may lead to frustration and discourage your progress.

Sustainability is crucial for long-term weight management. Avoid quick fixes or drastic measures that are not sustainable in the long run. Instead, focus on making gradual, healthy changes to your eating habits and physical activity levels. By adopting sustainable practices, you can establish a healthy lifestyle that supports your weight management goals and overall well-being.

2. Adopt a balanced and nutritious diet

Focus on consuming a variety of nutrient-dense foods such as fruits, vegetables, whole grains, lean proteins, and healthy fats. Limit the intake of processed foods, sugary drinks, and high-fat snacks. Portion control is also important, so pay attention to portion sizes and practice mindful eating.

3. Eat mindfully

Slow down while eating and pay attention to your body's hunger and fullness cues. Avoid distractions, such as TV or electronic devices, while eating to prevent overeating.

Practicing mindful eating is an effective strategy for weight management. By slowing down and paying attention to your eating experience, you can better tune in to your body's hunger and fullness cues. Avoiding distractions like television or electronic devices allows you to focus on the meal at hand and prevents mindless overeating.

When you eat mindfully, take the time to savor each bite, chew your food thoroughly, and appreciate the flavors and textures. This approach helps you become more aware of your body's signals of hunger and fullness, allowing you to eat in response to actual physiological needs rather than external cues.

By incorporating mindful eating into your routine, you can develop a healthier relationship with food, prevent overeating, and make more conscious food choices that support your weight management goals. It's a simple yet powerful technique that can make a significant difference in your eating habits and overall well-being.

4. Stay hydrated

Drink an adequate amount of water throughout the day. Sometimes, thirst can be mistaken for hunger, leading to unnecessary snacking. Staying hydrated is an important aspect of weight management. Drinking an adequate amount of water throughout the day helps maintain proper bodily functions and supports overall health. It also plays a role in managing hunger and preventing unnecessary snacking.

Sometimes, our bodies can confuse thirst with hunger, leading us to reach for food when what we really need is hydration. By staying well-hydrated, you can better differentiate between hunger and thirst cues, reducing the likelihood of mindless snacking or overeating.

Make it a habit to carry a water bottle with you and sip water throughout the day, even if you don't feel particularly thirsty. Aim to drink at least 8 cups (64 ounces) of water daily, or more if you engage in physical activity or are in a hot environment. Hydrating adequately can help support your weight management efforts and contribute to overall well-being.

5. Engage in regular physical activity

Incorporate both aerobic exercises (such as brisk walking, jogging, cycling, and swimming) and strength training exercises (such as weightlifting or resistance training) into your routine.

Aim for at least 150 minutes of moderate-intensity aerobic activity or 75 minutes of vigorous-intensity activity per week, along with strength training exercises twice a week.

6. Practice portion control

Be mindful of portion sizes and avoid oversized servings. Use smaller plates and bowls to help control portions visually. Pay attention to hunger and fullness cues to prevent overeating.

7. Monitor your food intake

Keeping a food diary or using a mobile app to track your food intake can help you become more aware of your eating habits and identify areas for improvement. It can also help you make more informed food choices and manage calorie intake.

8. Get enough sleep

Aim for 7-9 hours of quality sleep each night. Inadequate sleep can disrupt hunger and fullness hormones, leading to increased appetite and cravings.

9. Manage stress

Find healthy ways to cope with stress rather than turning to food for comfort. Engage in relaxation techniques such as deep breathing, meditation, or engaging in hobbies or activities you enjoy.

10. Seek support

Consider seeking support from healthcare professionals, such as registered dietitians or weight management specialists, who can provide guidance, support, and personalized strategies for weight management.

Remember, weight management is a long-term commitment to a healthy lifestyle rather than a short-term fix.

It's important to find strategies that work for you and to make gradual, sustainable changes. Consulting with healthcare professionals can provide personalized guidance based on your specific needs and circumstances.

Joint Protection Techniques

Joint protection techniques are strategies and practices aimed at reducing stress on the joints, preserving joint function, and minimizing pain for individuals with conditions such as arthritis or joint injuries.

Here are some joint protection techniques:

1. Maintain good posture

Practice proper body alignment and posture to minimize stress on the joints. When sitting, ensure that your back is straight, and use supportive chairs with good backrests. When standing, distribute your weight evenly on both feet.

2. Use assistive devices

Utilize assistive devices such as canes, crutches, walkers, or braces to provide support and stability to the joints, especially during weight-bearing activities.

3. Modify activities

Make adjustments to your daily activities to reduce joint stress. Avoid activities that involve repetitive joint movements or prolonged periods of joint stress. Break tasks into smaller, manageable parts, and take regular breaks to rest and change positions.

4. Lift and carry properly

When lifting heavy objects, use proper body mechanics. Bend at the knees and hips, not at the waist, and lift with the leg muscles rather than straining the joints.

Hold objects close to your body and avoid twisting or jerking motions.

5. Use ergonomic tools and equipment

Utilize tools and equipment designed with ergonomic principles to reduce joint strain. For example, use padded handles or grips on tools, or use larger handles for better grip and less joint stress.

6. Practice joint-friendly exercises

Engage in exercises that are low-impact and gentle on the joints, such as swimming, cycling, walking, or Tai chi, as these exercises can help improve joint flexibility, strength, and range of motion without placing excessive stress on the joints.

7. Apply heat or cold therapy

Use heat or cold therapy to manage joint pain and inflammation. Apply a heating pad, warm compress, or take a warm shower to help relax muscles and improve blood circulation. Cold packs or ice packs can be applied to reduce swelling and numb pain.

8. Manage weight

Maintaining a healthy weight reduces the load on weight-bearing joints, such as the knees and hips. By managing weight through a combination of healthy eating habits and regular exercise, you can alleviate stress on the joints.

9. Listen to your body

Pay attention to your body's signals and limitations. Rest when needed, and avoid overexertion or pushing through excessive pain. Pace yourself and find a balance between activity and rest to avoid exacerbating joint symptoms.

10. Seek professional guidance

Consult with healthcare professionals, such as physical therapists or occupational therapists, who can provide personalized guidance on joint protection techniques, recommend assistive devices, and design exercise programs tailored to your specific needs.

Remember, joint protection techniques may vary depending on the individual and the specific joint condition. It's important to consult with healthcare professionals to receive personalized advice and recommendations based on your unique circumstances.

Chapter 6

Assistive Devices and Adaptive Equipment

Osteoarthritis is a degenerative joint disease that commonly affects older adults. It can cause pain, stiffness, and reduced mobility, making everyday tasks challenging. However, there are various assistive devices and adaptive equipment available that can help individuals with osteoarthritis manage their symptoms and maintain their independence. These devices are designed to support and assist affected joints, reduce strain, and improve overall function.

Here are some examples:

1. Canes and Walkers

Canes provide stability and support while walking, reducing stress on the lower limbs and joints. Walkers offer even more support and can be beneficial for individuals with severe osteoarthritis or balance issues.

2. Knee Braces

Knee braces can provide stability, reduce pain, and offer support to the knee joint. They are available in various types, including sleeves, straps, and immobilizers, catering to different levels of knee support required.

3. Hand and Finger Splints

Hand and finger splints can alleviate pain and stiffness associated with osteoarthritis in the hands. They provide support, immobilization, and help maintain proper alignment of the affected joints.

4. Assistive Devices for Gripping and Grabbing

Tools such as reachers, long-handled shoe horns, and adaptive utensils can assist individuals with osteoarthritis in performing daily tasks that involve gripping, grabbing, or reaching objects.

5. Orthotic Shoe Inserts

Orthotic shoe inserts, also known as shoe orthotics or insoles, can provide cushioning, support, and alignment for the feet and lower limbs. They can help reduce joint pressure and improve walking comfort.

6. Bathroom Aids

Bathroom aids such as raised toilet seats, grab bars, shower chairs, and bath benches can enhance safety and accessibility in the bathroom, reducing the risk of falls and strain on affected joints.

7. Adaptive Tools for Activities of Daily Living (ADLs)

Various adaptive tools are available to assist with ADLs. For example, jar openers, button hooks, and zipper pulls can make dressing easier, while long-handled brushes and combs can assist with grooming.

8. Joint Protection Devices

Joint protection devices, such as compression sleeves, braces, or wraps, can provide support and stability to affected joints, reducing pain and minimizing further damage during physical activities.

9. Assistive Devices for Exercise

There are specialized assistive devices designed to facilitate exercise and physical activity for individuals with osteoarthritis. These may include stationary bikes, elliptical trainers with low impact, or resistance bands tailored for gentle joint movement.

10. Ergonomic Tools

Ergonomic tools and equipment, such as specially designed kitchen utensils or tools with padded handles, can help reduce strain on the joints while performing tasks like cooking, cleaning, or gardening.

11. Assistive Devices for Driving

Adaptations to vehicles, such as hand controls or steering wheel grips, can enable individuals with osteoarthritis to continue driving safely and comfortably.

12. Electric Mobility Scooters or Wheelchairs

For individuals with advanced osteoarthritis or limited mobility, electric mobility scooters or wheelchairs can provide independence and assist with transportation over longer distances.

13. Heat and Cold Therapy Devices

Heat and cold therapy devices, such as heating pads or cold packs, can help alleviate pain and inflammation associated with osteoarthritis. These can be used for targeted relief on specific joints.

14. Assistive Technology

Technological advancements have led to the development of various assistive devices, including voice-activated assistants, smart home systems, and mobile applications, which can help individuals with osteoarthritis manage their daily routines more efficiently.

15. Customized Assistive Devices

In some cases, individuals may require custom-made assistive devices tailored to their specific needs. These can be created by healthcare professionals or occupational therapists to address unique challenges posed by osteoarthritis.

It's important to note that while assistive devices and adaptive equipment can be helpful, it's advisable to consult with a healthcare professional or occupational therapist. They can assess individual needs, provide guidance on selecting the most appropriate devices, and offer additional strategies for managing osteoarthritis symptoms.

Understanding the Role of Assistive Devices

Assistive devices play a crucial role in enhancing the independence, mobility, and overall quality of life for individuals with disabilities or functional limitations. These devices are designed to compensate for impairments, promote accessibility, and enable individuals to perform various tasks and activities more easily.

Here are some key roles that assistive devices fulfill:

1. Enhancing Mobility

Assistive devices such as canes, walkers, crutches, and wheelchairs provide support and stability, allowing individuals with mobility impairments to move around independently. These devices reduce the risk of falls, improve balance, and increase overall mobility.

2. Promoting Accessibility

Assistive devices are essential in making environments more accessible for individuals with disabilities. Examples include ramps, stair lifts, and elevators, which ensure that people with mobility challenges can access buildings and navigate different levels.

3. Supporting Activities of Daily Living (ADLs)

Assistive devices aid individuals in performing everyday tasks. Devices such as dressing aids, adaptive utensils, reachers, and bathing aids enable people with disabilities or limited mobility to dress, eat, reach objects, and maintain personal hygiene independently.

4. Augmenting Communication

Communication devices like augmentative and alternative communication (AAC) devices, speech-generating devices, and text-to-speech software assist individuals with speech impairments in expressing themselves and interacting with others effectively.

5. Assisting Sensory Impairments

Assistive devices cater to individuals with sensory impairments. Hearing aids, cochlear implants, assistive listening devices, and visual aids (such as magnifiers or screen readers) enhance auditory or visual abilities, allowing people with hearing or vision loss to communicate and perceive the world around them.

6. Compensating for Cognitive Impairments

Individuals with cognitive impairments can benefit from assistive devices such as memory aids, electronic organizers, reminder systems, and assistive software that help with memory, organization, and task completion.

7. Reducing Pain and Discomfort

Assistive devices like orthotic shoe inserts, braces, splints, or cushions provide support and relieve pain associated with conditions such as arthritis, joint instability, or pressure sores.

8. Promoting Safety and Fall Prevention

Devices such as grab bars, bed rails, fall alarms, and motion sensors help create safer environments for individuals at risk of falls or injuries. These devices provide stability, assistance, and immediate alerts in case of accidents.

9. Enhancing Work and Productivity

Assistive devices designed for the workplace, such as ergonomic chairs, adjustable desks, speech recognition software, or specialized keyboards, enable individuals with disabilities to perform their job tasks effectively and comfortably.

10. Fostering Social Participation

Assistive devices can facilitate social engagement and participation. For example, mobility scooters, adapted bicycles, or sports wheelchairs enable individuals with mobility impairments to participate in recreational activities and community events.

It is important to note that the selection and use of assistive devices should be done in consultation with healthcare professionals, therapists, or specialists who can assess individual needs, provide training, and ensure proper fit and usage. Customization, training, and ongoing support are key to maximizing the benefits of assistive devices and promoting independence and well-being for individuals with disabilities or functional limitations.

Mobility Aids for Osteoarthritis

Mobility aids are essential for individuals with osteoarthritis to manage their symptoms, reduce pain, and improve their mobility. Here are some common mobility aids that can be beneficial for individuals with osteoarthritis:

1. Canes

Canes provide stability and support while walking, reducing strain on the lower limbs and joints. They can help alleviate pain and improve balance for individuals with osteoarthritis affecting the hips, knees, or ankles.

2. Walkers

Walkers offer more support than canes and are suitable for individuals with more severe osteoarthritis or balance issues. They provide stability and a wider base of support, helping individuals maintain their balance while walking.

3. Crutches

Crutches can be used by individuals who need significant support for their lower limbs. They are particularly helpful for those recovering from joint surgery or experiencing severe pain in one leg.

4. Knee Braces

Knee braces can provide stability, reduce pain, and offer support to the knee joint. They come in different types, including sleeves, straps, and immobilizers, catering to different levels of knee support required.

5. Mobility Scooters

Mobility scooters are battery-powered devices that provide independent mobility for individuals with osteoarthritis affecting their lower limbs or those who have difficulty walking long distances. They are especially useful for outdoor activities or navigating larger spaces.

6. Wheelchairs

Wheelchairs are suitable for individuals with more severe mobility limitations. They can be self-propelled or pushed by a caregiver, providing the option for both independent and assisted mobility.

7. Rollators

Rollators are wheeled walkers with a built-in seat and hand brakes. They offer stability, support, and the option to rest whenever needed. Rollators are particularly useful for individuals who experience fatigue or need intermittent breaks while walking.

It's important to consult with a healthcare professional or physical therapist to determine the most appropriate mobility aid for an individual's specific needs.

They can assess the individual's mobility, provide guidance on proper usage and fit, and recommend any additional modifications or accessories that may be beneficial.

Regular reassessment and adjustments to the mobility aid may also be necessary to ensure optimal support and functionality.

Chapter 7

Complementary and Alternative Therapies

Complementary and alternative therapies, often referred to as CAM therapies, are a diverse set of healthcare practices and treatment approaches that fall outside of conventional medical practices. These therapies are used alongside or in conjunction with conventional medical treatments to promote health, well-being, and symptom relief. They are often based on traditional healing practices, holistic philosophies, or alternative systems of medicine.

Here's a closer look at what complementary and alternative therapies entail:

1. Complementary Therapies

Complementary therapies are used alongside conventional medical treatments to enhance their effectiveness or manage side effects. These therapies are considered as a complement to standard medical care.

Examples of complementary therapies include:

- **Acupuncture**

This involves the insertion of thin needles into specific points on the body to promote pain relief and overall well-being.

- **Massage therapy**

The manipulation of soft tissues in the body to relieve muscle tension, reduce pain, and improve relaxation.

- **Yoga**

A mind-body practice that combines physical postures, breathing exercises, and meditation to improve flexibility, strength, and mental well-being.

- **Meditation**

A technique that involves focusing the mind and achieving a state of deep relaxation to promote stress reduction and mental clarity.

- **Herbal medicine**

The use of plant-based remedies, such as herbs, botanical extracts, and dietary supplements, for therapeutic purposes.

2. Alternative Therapies

Alternative therapies are used in place of conventional medical treatments. These therapies are often based on alternative systems of medicine or healing practices that differ from mainstream medical approaches.

Examples of alternative therapies include:

- **Homeopathy**

A system of medicine that uses highly diluted substances to stimulate the body's natural healing mechanisms.

- **Traditional Chinese Medicine (TCM)**

A holistic system of medicine that includes acupuncture, herbal medicine, dietary therapy, and various mind-body practices.

- **Ayurveda**

An ancient Indian system of medicine that focuses on achieving balance and harmony in the body through personalized lifestyle practices, herbal remedies, and dietary modifications.

- **Naturopathy**

A system of medicine that emphasizes natural healing, utilizing a combination of therapies such as nutrition, herbal medicine, lifestyle changes, and physical modalities.

It's important to note that while some complementary and alternative therapies have shown promise in certain conditions or for symptom management, their scientific evidence may vary. It is advisable to consult with healthcare professionals, including doctors and qualified practitioners of complementary and alternative therapies, to ensure safe and effective integration of these therapies with conventional medical treatments. They can provide guidance, assess individual needs, and help make informed decisions about incorporating these therapies into a comprehensive healthcare plan.

Acupuncture and Acupressure

Acupuncture and acupressure are two therapeutic techniques rooted in traditional Chinese medicine. Both practices involve stimulating specific points on the body to promote healing, relieve pain, and restore balance.

Here's an overview of acupuncture and acupressure:

1. Acupuncture

Acupuncture involves the insertion of thin, sterile needles into specific points on the body. These points are believed to be connected by pathways called meridians, through which vital energy, known as qi (pronounced "chee"), flows. By stimulating these points, acupuncture aims to balance the flow of qi and restore health.

During an acupuncture session, a trained practitioner will carefully select and insert needles into specific acupoints. The needles may be gently manipulated or stimulated by heat (moxibustion) or electrical impulses (electroacupuncture). The treatment is generally painless, and many people find it relaxing. Acupuncture is commonly used for pain management, stress reduction, digestive disorders, respiratory conditions, and various other health concerns.

2. Acupressure

Acupressure is a technique that involves applying pressure to specific acupoints on the body. Instead of using needles, acupressure relies on manual pressure, typically applied by fingers, thumbs, or specialized tools, to stimulate the points. By applying pressure, acupressure aims to promote the flow of qi, relieve tension, and restore balance in the body.

Acupressure can be performed by a trained practitioner or self-administered for self-care. It is often used to alleviate pain, reduce stress, promote relaxation, and improve overall well-being. Techniques such as tapping, kneading, or holding pressure on specific points are employed in acupressure.

Both acupuncture and acupressure are generally considered safe when performed by trained practitioners. They are used to address a wide range of conditions and symptoms, including musculoskeletal pain, headaches, nausea, insomnia, anxiety, and more. However, it's important to consult with a qualified healthcare professional or acupuncturist to determine if these therapies are suitable for individual needs and to ensure proper application and safety.

It's worth noting that scientific research on acupuncture and acupressure is ongoing, and their mechanisms of action are still being investigated. While some studies have shown positive results, more research is needed to fully understand their effectiveness and integration into mainstream healthcare practices.

Herbal Supplements and Natural Remedies

Herbal supplements and natural remedies refer to products derived from plants or natural sources that are used to promote health, prevent illness, or alleviate symptoms. These remedies have been used for centuries in various traditional healing systems around the world.

Here are some key points about herbal supplements and natural remedies:

1. Plant-Based Ingredients

Herbal supplements and natural remedies are typically made from plant materials such as leaves, flowers, roots, bark, or seeds. These ingredients contain various active compounds that are believed to have medicinal properties.

2. Traditional and Cultural Use

Many herbal remedies have a long history of traditional use in different cultures. Traditional systems of medicine, such as Ayurveda, Traditional Chinese Medicine (TCM), and Indigenous healing practices, have relied on herbal remedies as a primary form of treatment.

3. Active Constituents

Plants contain numerous chemical compounds that contribute to their therapeutic effects. These compounds may include alkaloids, flavonoids, terpenes, phenols, and more. Each plant species has a unique composition of these active constituents, which can influence their specific health benefits.

4. Common Uses

Herbal supplements and natural remedies are used for various purposes, including:

- Promoting general health and well-being
- Supporting immune function

- Aiding digestion and gastrointestinal health
- Managing symptoms of specific conditions, such as insomnia, anxiety, or menopause
- Providing relief from common ailments, such as colds, coughs, or headaches.

5. Safety and Quality

While herbal supplements and natural remedies are generally considered safe, it's important to exercise caution. Not all natural products are suitable for everyone, and they can interact with medications or cause adverse effects in certain individuals. It's crucial to consult with a healthcare professional before starting any new herbal supplement or natural remedy, especially if you have existing health conditions or are taking medications.

6. Standardization and Regulation

The quality and consistency of herbal supplements can vary, as they are not regulated as strictly as pharmaceutical drugs. It's advisable to choose products from reputable manufacturers that follow good manufacturing practices (GMP) and have undergone third-party testing for purity and potency.

7. Scientific Evidence

While traditional use and anecdotal evidence support the effectiveness of some herbal remedies, scientific research plays a critical role in evaluating their safety and efficacy. Some herbal supplements have been extensively studied, and their benefits have been supported by scientific evidence. However, for many herbal remedies, more research is needed to establish their effectiveness and understand their mechanisms of action.

8. Individual Variability

It's important to recognize that individual responses to herbal supplements and natural remedies can vary. What works for one person may not work for another, and it's essential to listen to your body and consult with a healthcare professional for personalized advice.

In summary, herbal supplements and natural remedies offer a diverse range of options for promoting health and well-being. However, it's crucial to approach them with caution, seek professional guidance, and be mindful of potential interactions or adverse effects. Integrating these remedies into a comprehensive healthcare plan should be done in collaboration with healthcare professionals who can provide guidance based on your individual needs and health circumstances.

Mind-Body Therapies for Pain Management

Mind-body therapies are a group of therapeutic approaches that recognize the interconnectedness of the mind and body and aim to promote healing, well-being, and pain management. These therapies utilize various techniques and practices to harness the mind's influence on physical health and alleviate pain.

Here are some mind-body therapies commonly used for pain management:

1. Meditation

Meditation involves focusing the mind and achieving a state of deep relaxation and mental clarity. It can help reduce pain perception, alleviate stress and anxiety, and improve overall well-being. Mindfulness meditation, in particular, teaches individuals to bring nonjudgmental awareness to their present moment experiences, including pain sensations, which can lead to increased pain acceptance and improved pain management.

2. Yoga

Yoga combines physical postures (asanas), breathing exercises (pranayama), and meditation to promote physical strength, flexibility, relaxation, and mental calmness. Regular practice of yoga can reduce pain, improve mobility, enhance body awareness, and provide a sense of overall well-being.

3. Tai Chi

Tai Chi is an ancient Chinese martial art that involves slow, gentle movements combined with deep breathing and focused attention. It promotes balance, relaxation, flexibility, and mind-body integration. Regular practice of Tai Chi has been shown to reduce pain, improve physical function, and enhance quality of life for individuals with chronic pain conditions.

4. Relaxation Techniques

Various relaxation techniques, such as progressive muscle relaxation, guided imagery, deep breathing exercises, and biofeedback, can help induce a state of deep relaxation, reduce muscle tension, and alleviate pain. These techniques promote relaxation responses in the body, counteracting the stress response associated with pain.

5. Cognitive-Behavioral Therapy (CBT)

CBT is a psychotherapeutic approach that focuses on identifying and changing negative thoughts and behaviors that contribute to pain perception and suffering. It helps individuals develop coping skills, manage stress, and improve their overall emotional well-being. CBT can be particularly effective in addressing chronic pain conditions by altering pain-related beliefs and improving pain self-management strategies.

6. Hypnotherapy

Hypnotherapy involves guided relaxation, focused attention, and suggestions to promote changes in perception, behavior, and experience. It can help individuals manage pain, reduce anxiety, enhance relaxation, and improve overall well-being. Hypnotherapy can be used in conjunction with other pain management strategies.

7. Biofield Therapies

Biofield therapies, such as Reiki, Healing Touch, and Therapeutic Touch, work with the energy fields around the body to promote relaxation, balance, and healing. These therapies involve the gentle placement of hands or non-contact approaches to influence the flow of energy and facilitate the body's self-healing abilities. While the scientific evidence for biofield therapies is limited, some individuals find them beneficial for pain relief and relaxation.

8. Mindfulness-Based Stress Reduction (MBSR)

MBSR is a program that combines mindfulness meditation, body awareness, and yoga practices to help individuals manage stress, pain, and illness. It teaches participants to cultivate non-judgmental awareness of their thoughts, emotions, and bodily sensations, promoting acceptance and self-care.

9. Guided Imagery

Guided imagery involves using the power of imagination and visualization to evoke positive mental images and sensations. It can help individuals reduce pain, manage stress, and promote relaxation by creating a calming and pleasant mental state. During guided imagery, a person typically listens to a recorded script or receives verbal guidance from a practitioner or therapist.

The guidance directs the individual to imagine specific sensory details, such as sights, sounds, smells, and physical sensations that evoke a peaceful and tranquil environment. This might involve visualizing oneself in a serene natural setting, such as a beach or a forest, or imagining a specific scenario that elicits feelings of relaxation and happiness.

The key idea behind guided imagery is that the mind and body are interconnected, and by creating positive mental images, individuals can positively influence their physical and emotional states. Research suggests that practicing guided imagery regularly can help reduce anxiety, alleviate pain, enhance immune function, improve sleep quality, and enhance overall well-being.

10. Breathwork

Breathwork techniques, such as deep breathing exercises, diaphragmatic breathing, and alternate nostril breathing, focus on conscious control of the breath. These techniques can help regulate the autonomic nervous system, reduce stress, promote relaxation, and alleviate pain.

11. Art Therapy

Art therapy involves using creative processes, such as painting, drawing, or sculpting, as a means of expression and self-discovery. It can be used to explore emotions related to pain, reduce stress, and promote psychological well-being.

12. Music Therapy

Music therapy utilizes the therapeutic properties of music to support pain management and emotional well-being. Listening to or actively engaging in music can help reduce pain perception, promote relaxation, and improve mood.

It's important to note that mind-body therapies are typically used as part of a comprehensive pain management plan and should be integrated with other appropriate medical treatments and interventions. Consulting with healthcare professionals and seeking guidance from trained practitioners in these therapies can help ensure their safe and effective use in managing pain and promoting overall well-being.

Chapter 8

Diet and Nutrition for Osteoarthritis

Diet and nutrition play a significant role in managing osteoarthritis and promoting joint health. While there is no specific diet that can cure osteoarthritis, adopting a healthy eating plan can help reduce inflammation, support weight management, and provide essential nutrients for joint health.

Here are some dietary recommendations for osteoarthritis:

1. Maintaining a Healthy Weight

Excess weight puts additional stress on the joints, particularly the knees, hips, and spine. Losing weight or maintaining a healthy weight can help reduce pain and slow down the progression of osteoarthritis. A balanced, calorie-controlled diet that includes whole foods, fruits, vegetables, lean proteins, and healthy fats can support weight management.

2. Consume Anti-inflammatory Foods

Chronic inflammation plays a role in the progression of osteoarthritis. Including anti-inflammatory foods in your diet can help reduce inflammation and alleviate symptoms. Examples of anti-inflammatory foods include fatty fish (such as salmon and sardines), walnuts, flaxseeds, chia seeds, olive oil, green leafy vegetables, berries, turmeric, ginger, and green tea.

3. Incorporate Omega-3 Fatty Acids

Omega-3 fatty acids have anti-inflammatory properties and may help reduce joint pain and stiffness in osteoarthritis. Good sources of omega-3 fatty acids include fatty fish (such as salmon, mackerel, and trout), walnuts, flaxseeds, chia seeds, and hemp seeds. If necessary, omega-3 supplements can be considered, but it's advisable to consult with a healthcare professional first.

4. Choose Nutrient-Dense Foods

Opt for a diet rich in nutrient-dense foods to support overall health and provide essential vitamins and minerals for joint health. Include a variety of fruits, vegetables, whole grains, lean proteins (such as poultry, fish, legumes, and tofu), nuts, and seeds in your meals. These foods provide antioxidants, vitamins (particularly vitamins C and D), minerals (such as calcium and magnesium), and other nutrients important for maintaining healthy joints.

5. Limit Processed Foods and Added Sugars

Processed foods, fast food, sugary beverages, and snacks high in added sugars can promote inflammation and contribute to weight gain. Limiting the consumption of these foods can help manage inflammation and maintain a healthy weight. Instead, opt for whole, minimally processed foods whenever possible.

6. Stay Hydrated

Proper hydration is important for joint health. Drinking an adequate amount of water throughout the day helps keep the joints lubricated and supports the overall functioning of the body. Limit the consumption of sugary drinks and opt for water, herbal tea, or infused water instead.

7. Consider Supplements

Some individuals may benefit from specific supplements for joint health. Glucosamine and chondroitin sulfate are commonly used to support joint cartilage health, although the scientific evidence is mixed. It's advisable to consult with a healthcare professional before starting any new supplements to ensure their safety and suitability for your specific condition.

8. Limit Saturated and Trans Fats

High intake of saturated and trans fats found in fried foods, processed snacks, and fatty meats may promote inflammation. Choose healthier fats, such as monounsaturated fats found in olive oil and avocados, and polyunsaturated fats found in nuts, seeds, and fatty fish.

9. Increase Fiber Intake

Consuming an adequate amount of dietary fiber from whole grains, fruits, vegetables, and legumes can help support digestive health, maintain a healthy weight, and potentially reduce inflammation.

10. Moderate Alcohol Consumption

Excessive alcohol intake can contribute to inflammation and may negatively affect joint health. If you choose to drink alcohol, do so in moderation, following the guidelines provided by healthcare professionals.

11. Limit Added Salt

High sodium intake can lead to water retention and may contribute to joint inflammation. Limit your intake of processed and packaged foods, as they often contain high levels of added salt. Instead, season your meals with herbs, spices, and natural flavorings.

12. Individualize Your Diet

Remember that everyone's nutritional needs are unique, and it's important to consider your overall health, medical conditions, and potential medication interactions when making dietary choices. Working with a registered dietitian can help you develop a personalized eating plan that addresses your specific needs and goals.

13. Include Antioxidant-Rich Foods

Antioxidants help protect the body against oxidative stress and inflammation. Include a variety of colorful fruits and vegetables in your diet, such as berries, leafy greens, citrus fruits, and cruciferous vegetables like broccoli and cauliflower.

14. Consume Adequate Calcium

Calcium is important for maintaining strong bones and may help slow the progression of osteoarthritis. Include calcium-rich foods in your diet, such as dairy products (if tolerated), fortified plant-based milk, leafy greens, tofu, and almonds. If needed, consider calcium supplements, but consult with a healthcare professional first.

15. Vitamin D

Adequate vitamin D levels are crucial for bone health. Get regular exposure to sunlight and include vitamin D-rich foods in your diet, such as fatty fish, fortified dairy products, egg yolks, and mushrooms. If necessary, vitamin D supplements may be recommended, particularly for individuals with limited sun exposure or low levels.

16. Herbal Remedies

Some herbal remedies, such as ginger and turmeric, have anti-inflammatory properties and may help reduce pain and inflammation in osteoarthritis. However, it's important to consult with a healthcare professional before using herbal remedies, as they can interact with medications or have potential side effects.

17. Hyaluronic Acid

Hyaluronic acid supplements or injections may be recommended by healthcare professionals for individuals with osteoarthritis. Hyaluronic acid is a component of joint fluid and may help improve joint lubrication and reduce pain. Talk to your healthcare provider to determine if hyaluronic acid is suitable for you.

18. Avoid Food Sensitivities

Some individuals may experience increased joint pain or inflammation due to specific food sensitivities or allergies. If you suspect certain foods may be exacerbating your symptoms, consider keeping a food diary and working with a healthcare professional to identify and eliminate potential triggers.

Remember, everyone's nutritional needs are unique, and it's important to consult with a healthcare professional or a registered dietitian to develop a personalized dietary plan that takes into account your specific health needs, medical conditions, and potential medication interactions. They can provide guidance tailored to your individual circumstances and help you make informed choices to support your overall well-being and manage osteoarthritis effectively.

Anti-inflammatory Foods and Nutrients

Anti-inflammatory foods and nutrients have been shown to help reduce inflammation in the body and support overall health. Including these foods in your diet can be beneficial for managing conditions such as osteoarthritis.

Here are some examples of anti-inflammatory foods and nutrients:

1. **Fatty Fish**

Fatty fish such as salmon, mackerel, sardines, and trout are rich in omega-3 fatty acids. Omega-3s have been shown to reduce inflammation and may help alleviate symptoms of joint pain and stiffness.

2. **Berries**

Berries like blueberries, strawberries, raspberries, and blackberries are packed with antioxidants, which help combat inflammation and protect cells from damage. They are also rich in fiber and vitamins.

3. **Leafy Green Vegetables**

Leafy greens such as spinach, kale, and Swiss chard are excellent sources of vitamins, minerals, and antioxidants. They contain compounds that help reduce inflammation and support overall health.

4. **Nuts and Seeds**

Almonds, walnuts, flaxseeds, and chia seeds are rich in healthy fats, fiber, and antioxidants. They provide anti-inflammatory benefits and can be incorporated into meals, snacks, or as toppings for salads and yogurt.

5. **Turmeric**

Turmeric is a spice that contains a compound called curcumin, which has potent anti-inflammatory properties. Adding turmeric to your meals or using it in teas and smoothies can help reduce inflammation. Curcumin has been studied for its potential to reduce inflammation in various conditions, including osteoarthritis.

6. **Ginger**

Ginger has been used for centuries for its medicinal properties, including anti-inflammatory effects. It can be used in cooking, added to teas, or consumed in supplement form to help reduce inflammation.

7. Olive Oil

Olive oil is a healthy fat that contains monounsaturated fatty acids and antioxidants. It has been shown to have anti-inflammatory effects and is a staple of the Mediterranean diet.

8. Green Tea

Green tea is rich in antioxidants called catechins, which have anti-inflammatory properties. Drinking green tea regularly may help reduce inflammation and promote overall health.

9. Tomatoes

Tomatoes are rich in lycopene, an antioxidant with anti-inflammatory properties. Cooking tomatoes or consuming them with a source of healthy fat, like olive oil, can enhance the absorption of lycopene.

10. Dark Chocolate

Dark chocolate with a high percentage of cocoa (70% or higher) contains flavonoids that have anti-inflammatory effects. Moderation is key, as dark chocolate is also calorie-dense.

11. Spices

Certain spices like cinnamon, cayenne pepper, and cloves have been shown to have anti-inflammatory properties. Adding them to your meals can provide both flavor and potential health benefits.

12. Garlic

Garlic has been recognized for its medicinal properties for centuries. It contains sulfur compounds that have anti-inflammatory effects. Incorporating garlic into your meals can provide both flavor and potential health benefits.

13. Onions

Onions, like garlic, contain sulfur compounds that have anti-inflammatory properties. They can be used in various dishes to add flavor and provide potential health benefits.

14. Cherries

Cherries, especially tart cherries, are rich in antioxidants called anthocyanins. These compounds have been shown to have anti-inflammatory effects. Consuming cherries or tart cherry juice may help reduce inflammation and alleviate symptoms of osteoarthritis.

15. Pineapple

Pineapple contains an enzyme called bromelain, which has anti-inflammatory properties. Bromelain may help reduce inflammation and promote joint health. Fresh pineapple or pineapple juice can be included in the diet to reap these potential benefits.

16. Cruciferous Vegetables:

Vegetables like broccoli, cauliflower, cabbage, and Brussels sprouts are part of the cruciferous family and are known for their anti-inflammatory properties. They are rich in antioxidants, fiber, and other beneficial compounds.

17. Bell Peppers

Bell peppers, particularly red and yellow varieties, are excellent sources of vitamin C and antioxidants. Vitamin C plays a crucial role in collagen synthesis, which is important for maintaining healthy joints.

18. Extra Virgin Olive Oil

Extra virgin olive oil is a healthy fat rich in monounsaturated fatty acids and antioxidants. It has been associated with reduced inflammation and improved joint health. It is best used in its raw form or for low-heat cooking.

19. Green Leafy Herbs:

Herbs like basil, parsley, and cilantro not only add flavor to meals but also provide anti-inflammatory benefits. They are rich in vitamins, minerals, and antioxidants that support overall health.

Incorporating these anti-inflammatory foods into a balanced diet can help reduce inflammation, support joint health, and promote overall well-being.

It's important to note that dietary changes alone may not be sufficient to manage osteoarthritis, and they should be combined with other appropriate medical treatments and lifestyle modifications. Consulting with a healthcare professional or registered dietitian can help create a personalized eating plan that meets your specific needs.

Supplements for Joint Health

Supplements are products that are designed to supplement or enhance the intake of nutrients in the diet. They come in various forms such as capsules, tablets, powders, liquids, or gummies. Supplements are intended to provide additional vitamins, minerals, herbs, botanicals, amino acids, or other beneficial substances that may be lacking in the diet or required in higher amounts for certain individuals.

There are several supplements that are commonly used to support joint health. Here are some of the most popular ones:

1. Glucosamine

Glucosamine is a natural compound found in healthy cartilage. It is commonly used to help support joint health and may help reduce joint pain and stiffness.

2. Chondroitin

Chondroitin is another compound found in cartilage. It works in combination with glucosamine to support joint health and may help reduce joint pain and improve joint function.

3. MSM (Methylsulfonylmethane)

MSM is a sulfur compound that is believed to have anti-inflammatory properties. It is often used to relieve joint pain and improve joint flexibility.

4. Omega-3 fatty acids

Omega-3 fatty acids, found in fish oil, are known for their anti-inflammatory properties. They can help reduce inflammation in the joints and may alleviate joint pain and stiffness.

5. Turmeric

Turmeric contains a compound called curcumin, which has powerful anti-inflammatory properties. It is often used to help reduce joint pain and inflammation.

6. Boswellia

Boswellia is an herbal supplement derived from the Boswellia serrata tree. It has been traditionally used in Ayurvedic medicine to support joint health and reduce inflammation.

7. Ginge

Ginger has anti-inflammatory properties and may help reduce joint pain and swelling. It can be consumed as a supplement or added to meals and beverages.

8. Vitamin D

Vitamin D plays a role in maintaining healthy bones and joints. Low levels of vitamin D have been associated with an increased risk of joint pain and arthritis.

9. Calcium

Calcium is important for maintaining strong bones and may help support joint health. It is commonly found in dairy products, leafy greens, and fortified foods.

It's important to note that while these supplements are widely used and have shown potential benefits for joint health, individual results may vary. It's always a good idea to consult with a healthcare professional before starting any new supplement regimen, especially if you have any underlying health conditions or are taking other medications.

Creating a Balanced Osteoarthritis Diet Plan

A balanced diet can play a crucial role in managing osteoarthritis and supporting joint health. Here is a general outline of a balanced osteoarthritis diet plan:

1. Include a variety of fruits and vegetables

Aim for a colorful array of fruits and vegetables, as they are rich in antioxidants and anti-inflammatory compounds. Include berries, citrus fruits, leafy greens, broccoli, carrots, and sweet potatoes.

2. Choose whole grains

Opt for whole grains like brown rice, quinoa, whole wheat bread, and whole grain pasta. They provide fiber and essential nutrients while promoting satiety.

3. Consume lean protein

Include lean sources of protein in your diet such as skinless poultry, fish (salmon, trout, sardines), legumes (beans, lentils), and tofu. Protein is essential for muscle health and repair.

4. Incorporate healthy fats

Include sources of healthy fats like avocados, nuts, seeds, and olive oil. Omega-3 fatty acids found in fatty fish (salmon, mackerel) and flaxseeds may have anti-inflammatory properties.

5. Limit saturated and trans fats

Minimize the consumption of saturated and trans fats found in fried foods, fatty meats, processed snacks, and baked goods. These fats may promote inflammation and increase the risk of chronic diseases.

6. Emphasize low-fat dairy or alternatives

Choose low-fat dairy products like milk, yogurt, and cheese. If you prefer non-dairy options, select fortified plant-based alternatives such as almond milk or soy milk.

7. Watch your portion sizes

Maintaining a healthy weight is important for managing osteoarthritis. Be mindful of portion sizes to prevent excess calorie intake, which can contribute to weight gain and joint stress.

8. Stay hydrated

Drink plenty of water throughout the day to keep your body hydrated and support joint function.

9. Limit processed foods and added sugars

Minimize the intake of processed foods, sugary snacks, sodas, and sugary beverages, as they can contribute to inflammation and weight gain.

10. Consider supplements

Consult with a healthcare professional to determine if any specific supplements may be beneficial for your osteoarthritis management, such as omega-3 fatty acids, glucosamine, or vitamin D.

Remember, it's important to personalize your diet plan according to your specific needs and preferences. Consulting with a registered dietitian can provide you with personalized guidance and help you create a diet plan tailored to your individual requirements.

Chapter 9

Emotional Well-being and Support

Emotional well-being and support refer to the state of one's overall emotional health and having access to the necessary resources, strategies, and social support systems to address and maintain optimal emotional well-being. It involves effectively managing and navigating emotions, coping with stress, maintaining positive relationships, and seeking support when needed.

Emotional well-being and support are important aspects of managing osteoarthritis and maintaining overall health. Dealing with a chronic condition like osteoarthritis can bring various emotional challenges, including stress, anxiety, depression, and frustration.

Here are some strategies to promote emotional well-being and seek support when living with osteoarthritis:

1. Self-awareness

Take the time to understand and acknowledge your emotions related to osteoarthritis. Recognize any feelings of frustration, sadness, or anxiety that may arise due to the challenges posed by the condition. Being aware of your emotions allows you to address them and seek appropriate support.

2. Open communication

Share your feelings and experiences with trusted family members, friends, or a support group. Communicating about your challenges and emotions can help you feel understood and supported. It also allows your loved ones to better understand what you're going through.

3. Seek professional support

Consider seeking help from mental health professionals, such as therapists or counselors, who specialize in chronic illness or pain management. They can provide valuable guidance and coping strategies to manage the emotional impact of osteoarthritis.

4. Join support groups

Connect with others who are also living with osteoarthritis by joining support groups, either in-person or online. These groups provide a platform for sharing experiences, exchanging tips and strategies, and receiving emotional support from individuals who truly understand the challenges of living with the condition.

5. Engage in stress-reducing activities

Engaging in stress-management techniques can promote emotional well-being. Practices like meditation, deep breathing exercises, mindfulness, or engaging in hobbies and activities you enjoy can help reduce stress and enhance your overall emotional health.

6. Maintain a positive mindset

Cultivate a positive outlook by focusing on the aspects of life that bring you joy and fulfillment. Celebrate small victories and achievements, and practice gratitude for the things you can still do despite the challenges posed by osteoarthritis.

7. Adapt and modify activities

Find ways to adapt your daily activities to accommodate your condition. This may involve using assistive devices, pacing yourself, and seeking alternative ways to engage in activities you enjoy. Making these adjustments can help maintain a sense of independence and contribute to your emotional well-being.

8. Practice self-care

Prioritize self-care activities that promote your physical, emotional, and mental well-being. This may include getting enough sleep, eating a balanced diet, engaging in regular physical activity within your capabilities, and engaging in activities that bring you joy and relaxation.

9. Educate yourself

Gain knowledge about osteoarthritis, its management, and treatment options. Understanding the condition can help alleviate anxiety and empower you to make informed decisions about your health.

10. Be patient and kind to yourself

Living with osteoarthritis can be challenging, so it's important to practice self-compassion and be patient with yourself. Remember to pace yourself, listen to your body, and prioritize self-care as you navigate the emotional aspects of the condition.

Remember that seeking emotional well-being and support is an ongoing process. Be open to trying different strategies and approaches, and don't hesitate to reach out for support when needed. Your emotional well-being is an important aspect of managing osteoarthritis and living a fulfilling life.

Coping with the Emotional Impact of Osteoarthritis

Coping with the emotional impact of osteoarthritis can be challenging, as the condition can have a significant impact on daily life, mobility, and overall well-being.

Here are some strategies to help cope with the emotional aspects of osteoarthritis:

1. Acknowledge your emotions

Recognize and validate your feelings about having osteoarthritis. It's normal to feel frustrated, sad, angry, or anxious about the changes and limitations the condition brings. Allow yourself to experience and express these emotions.

2. Educate yourself

Learn more about osteoarthritis to better understand the condition, its progression, and available management options. Knowledge can help reduce uncertainty and empower you to make informed decisions about your health.

3. Build a support system

Surround yourself with a supportive network of family, friends, or support groups who can provide understanding, empathy, and encouragement. Sharing your experiences and challenges with others who can relate can be comforting and provide a sense of validation.

4. Communicate with your healthcare team

Maintain open and honest communication with your healthcare provider. Share your emotional concerns and challenges related to osteoarthritis. They can offer guidance, support, and referrals to other professionals if needed.

5. Practice self-care

Engage in activities that promote self-care and well-being. This can include engaging in hobbies, practicing relaxation techniques, getting regular exercise (within the limits set by your healthcare provider), maintaining a balanced diet, and getting adequate rest and sleep.

6. Manage pain effectively

Seek appropriate pain management strategies to alleviate physical discomfort and minimize its impact on your emotional well-being. This may involve medication, physical therapy, hot/cold therapy, or other methods recommended by your healthcare provider.

7. Adapt and modify activities

Find ways to adapt and modify your daily activities to accommodate your condition. This can help you maintain a sense of independence and engagement in meaningful activities, reducing the emotional impact of limitations.

8. Seek professional help if needed

If you're experiencing significant emotional distress, consider seeking support from a mental health professional. They can provide guidance, coping strategies, and support tailored to your specific needs.

9. Practice stress management techniques

Engage in stress-reducing activities such as deep breathing exercises, meditation, mindfulness, or engaging in hobbies that promote relaxation and joy.

10. Focus on the positives

Cultivate a positive mindset by focusing on what you can do rather than what you can't. Celebrate small victories and achievements, and practice gratitude for the aspects of life that bring joy and fulfillment.

Remember, coping with the emotional impact of osteoarthritis is a personal journey, and different strategies may work for different individuals. Be patient with yourself, practice self-compassion, and seek support when needed.

Seeking Support from Family and Friends

Seeking support from family and friends can be incredibly beneficial when coping with the emotional impact of osteoarthritis. Here are some ways you can involve your loved ones in your support system:

1. **Open communication**

Share your feelings, challenges, and experiences with your family and friends. Let them know how osteoarthritis affects you both physically and emotionally. Open communication can foster understanding and empathy.

2. **Educate them about osteoarthritis**

Provide information about the condition, its symptoms, limitations, and treatment options. Help them understand what you're going through so they can offer appropriate support.

3. **Express your needs**

Clearly communicate your needs to your loved ones. Let them know what kind of support you would appreciate, whether it's assistance with daily tasks, accompaniment to medical appointments, or simply lending a listening ear.

4. **Encourage active participation**

Involve your family and friends in your healthcare journey. If appropriate, invite them to attend medical appointments or therapy sessions with you. This can help them understand your condition better and foster a sense of shared responsibility.

5. **Seek practical assistance**

Don't hesitate to ask for help with practical tasks that may be challenging due to your condition. It could be household chores, grocery shopping, or running errands. Loved ones who are willing to lend a helping hand can alleviate some of your physical and emotional burdens.

6. Emotional support

Share your emotions and feelings with your family and friends. Expressing your concerns, fears, or frustrations can provide relief and help them understand what you're going through. Having a compassionate listener can be incredibly comforting.

7. Participate in activities together

Engage in activities that you can enjoy with your loved ones, even if they need to be modified to accommodate your condition. It could be going for a walk, watching a movie, or having a meal together. Social connections and shared experiences can uplift your spirits.

8. Join support groups together

Consider attending support groups or educational sessions about osteoarthritis together. This can help your loved ones gain insight, learn coping strategies, and connect with others who may be going through similar experiences.

9. Practice empathy and patience

Remember that your loved ones may also need time to adjust and understand the impact of osteoarthritis on your life. Encourage open dialogue and foster an environment of empathy and patience for each other.

10. Express gratitude

Show appreciation for the support and understanding your family and friends provide. Expressing gratitude can strengthen your relationships and create a positive support network.

Remember, not everyone may fully understand what you're going through, but involving your loved ones and seeking their support can make a significant difference in managing the emotional impact of osteoarthritis.

Joining Osteoarthritis Support Groups

Joining osteoarthritis support groups can be a valuable resource for coping with the condition and connecting with others who understand your experiences. These groups provide a safe space to share your challenges, learn from others, and gain emotional support.

When seeking and joining osteoarthritis support groups, it is important to begin by researching available options in your local community or online. You can reach out to hospitals, clinics, community centers, or online platforms dedicated to arthritis or chronic conditions to gather information about support group options. This research will help you identify groups that align with your needs and preferences.

Consider the format of the support group. Support groups can take various formats, such as in-person meetings, online forums, or virtual meetings. Evaluate which format would be most convenient and comfortable for you to participate in regularly. If you prefer face-to-face interactions, you may opt for an in-person group. If you have limitations that make attending physical meetings difficult, online forums or virtual meetings may be more suitable.

Once you have chosen a support group, attend a meeting or join an online group. This initial participation will allow you to assess if the group is a good fit for you. Observe how the members interact, the level of support and understanding they provide, and the topics discussed. It is important to feel comfortable and accepted in the group to fully benefit from the support.

When participating in the support group, engage actively by sharing your experiences, asking questions, and offering support to others. Active participation can be therapeutic and create a sense of community. By sharing your journey and challenges, you not only receive support but also provide support to others going through similar experiences.

One of the advantages of support groups is the opportunity to learn from others. Take advantage of the collective knowledge and experiences of the group members to learn new coping mechanisms, treatment options, and self-care strategies. Support groups often provide a platform for exchanging information, tips, and resources related to managing osteoarthritis.

Seek emotional support within the group. Osteoarthritis can bring about emotional challenges, and sharing these with others who understand can be incredibly comforting. Whether it's expressing frustrations, fears, or celebrating small victories, the support group can provide a space for you to share and receive empathy.

It is important to respect boundaries and confidentiality within the support group. Establish trust and maintain confidentiality by honoring the personal stories and information shared by others. Respect the guidelines and rules established by the group to create a safe and supportive environment.

In summary, joining osteoarthritis support groups can provide valuable emotional support, knowledge sharing, and a sense of community. Through active participation and engagement, you can gain support, learn coping strategies, and develop meaningful connections with others facing similar challenges.

Chapter 10

Advanced Osteoarthritis

Advanced osteoarthritis refers to the later stages of osteoarthritis, a degenerative joint disease that commonly affects weight-bearing joints such as the knees, hips, and spine. In advanced stages, the condition has progressed and can significantly impact a person's joint function, mobility, and overall quality of life.

One of the key characteristics of advanced osteoarthritis is joint damage. The cartilage that normally cushions the joints becomes significantly worn down or damaged. As a result, the bones in the affected joint may start rubbing against each other, leading to pain, inflammation, and joint deformities.

The pain experienced in advanced osteoarthritis is often severe and persistent. It may worsen during movement or weight-bearing activities and can significantly limit a person's ability to perform daily tasks or engage in physical activities they once enjoyed. The pain can have a significant impact on a person's quality of life and overall well-being.

Loss of joint function is another notable feature of advanced osteoarthritis. As the joint damage progresses, individuals may experience joint stiffness, a decreased range of motion, and difficulty in performing movements or bearing weight. Simple tasks like walking, bending, or climbing stairs can become challenging and painful.

Joint deformities are common in advanced osteoarthritis. Bone spurs, also known as osteophytes, can develop around the joint edges, and joint misalignment can occur. These changes further contribute to pain, instability, and reduced joint function. Deformities can affect the overall alignment and mechanics of the joint, leading to further complications and limitations.

The impaired mobility caused by advanced osteoarthritis can have a significant impact on a person's independence and quality of life. It may require the use of assistive devices such as canes, walkers, or wheelchairs to aid in mobility and reduce joint stress. Mobility challenges can also lead to social isolation and decreased participation in activities, which can impact emotional well-being.

It is important for individuals with advanced osteoarthritis to work closely with healthcare professionals to manage their condition effectively. Treatment options may include a combination of pain management techniques, physical therapy, assistive devices, and, in severe cases, surgical interventions like joint replacement.

It is worth noting that while advanced osteoarthritis presents significant challenges, there are ways to manage the condition and improve quality of life. Seeking appropriate medical care, adopting healthy lifestyle habits, and exploring pain management strategies can all contribute to better joint function, reduced pain, and improved overall well-being.

Surgical Options for Advanced Osteoarthritis

Surgical options are available for individuals with advanced osteoarthritis when conservative treatments have not provided sufficient relief or when joint damage is severe. These surgical interventions aim to reduce pain, improve joint function, and enhance overall quality of life.

Here are some common surgical options for advanced osteoarthritis:

1. Joint replacement surgery

Joint replacement, also known as arthroplasty, is a commonly performed surgical procedure for advanced osteoarthritis. It involves removing the damaged joint surfaces and replacing them with artificial components made of metal, plastic, or ceramic. The most common joint replacements are total hip replacement, total knee replacement, and total shoulder replacement. Joint replacement surgery can significantly reduce pain, improve joint mobility, and enhance overall function.

2. Partial joint replacement

In some cases, when only one part of the joint is severely affected, a partial joint replacement may be recommended. This procedure involves replacing only the damaged portion of the joint, while preserving the healthy portions. Examples include unicompartmental knee replacement or hemiarthroplasty of the hip.

3. Joint fusion (arthrodesis)

Joint fusion is a surgical procedure where the damaged joint surfaces are removed and the bones on either side of the joint are fused together. This eliminates movement at the joint and can provide pain relief. Joint fusion is typically used for smaller joints such as the wrist, ankle, or fingers.

4. Osteotomy

Osteotomy is a procedure that involves reshaping or repositioning the bones around the affected joint to relieve pain and improve alignment. It is commonly performed in the knee joint to shift the weight-bearing forces to a healthier part of the joint.

5. Cartilage transplantation

In some cases, particularly for smaller areas of cartilage damage, cartilage transplantation procedures may be considered. This involves taking healthy cartilage tissue from one part of the body and transplanting it to the damaged area. These procedures are often performed on the knee joint.

6. Arthroscopy

Arthroscopy is a minimally invasive surgical procedure that uses a small camera and specialized instruments to visualize and treat joint conditions. It can be used to remove loose cartilage or bone fragments, repair or remove damaged tissues, and smooth out irregular joint surfaces. Arthroscopy is commonly performed in the knee joint.

7. Synovectomy

Synovectomy is a surgical procedure that involves removing the inflamed synovial tissue lining the joint. It is typically performed in cases where the synovium becomes thickened and causes pain and inflammation. Synovectomy can help alleviate symptoms and slow down the progression of joint damage.

8. Resurfacing procedures

In certain cases, joint resurfacing procedures may be an option. These procedures involve smoothing out the damaged joint surfaces without completely replacing the joint. They are often performed in younger patients with specific joint conditions or preferences.

It's important to note that the suitability of surgical options for advanced osteoarthritis varies depending on factors such as the location and severity of joint damage, overall health, and individual preferences. A thorough evaluation by a healthcare professional specializing in orthopedic surgery is necessary to determine the most appropriate surgical approach for each individual.

Recovery and rehabilitation following surgery are crucial for optimal outcomes. Physical therapy and rehabilitation programs are often recommended to help regain joint function, rebuild strength, and improve mobility. Post-operative care, including pain management, wound care, and following prescribed rehabilitation protocols, is essential for a successful recovery.

As with any surgical procedure, there are potential risks and complications associated with surgical interventions for advanced osteoarthritis. These can include infection, blood clots, nerve damage, and implant-related issues. It's important to discuss these risks with the healthcare team and ensure that all concerns and questions are addressed before making a decision to proceed with surgery.

Overall, surgical options for advanced osteoarthritis can provide significant relief and improve quality of life for individuals with severe joint damage. However, the decision to undergo surgery should be made in collaboration with healthcare professionals, as they will evaluate the severity of the condition, consider the individual's overall health, and discuss the potential risks and benefits of each surgical option. Rehabilitation and post-operative care are also essential to ensure optimal recovery and long-term success of the surgical intervention.

Joint Replacement Surgery: Benefits and Risks

Joint replacement surgery, also known as arthroplasty, is a commonly performed surgical procedure for individuals with advanced joint conditions, including severe osteoarthritis. It involves removing the damaged joint surfaces and replacing them with artificial components made of metal, plastic, or ceramic. Here are some benefits and risks associated with joint replacement surgery:

Benefits of Joint Replacement Surgery

1. **Pain relief**

One of the primary goals of joint replacement surgery is to alleviate chronic joint pain. The damaged joint surfaces, which are a significant source of pain, are replaced with prosthetic components that function smoothly, reducing or eliminating pain.

2. Improved joint function

Joint replacement surgery can significantly improve joint function, allowing individuals to regain mobility and engage in activities they may have previously been unable to perform. It can restore range of motion, stability, and strength to the affected joint.

3. Enhanced quality of life

Reduced pain and improved joint function can greatly enhance overall quality of life. Joint replacement surgery can enable individuals to resume daily activities, participate in hobbies, and enjoy a more active and independent lifestyle.

4. Long-lasting results

Joint replacements are designed to be durable and can last for many years. While the longevity of the implant can vary depending on factors such as patient age, activity level, and implant type, most individuals can expect their joint replacement to provide long-lasting relief for a considerable period.

Risks of Joint Replacement Surgery

1. Infection

Infection is a potential risk with any surgical procedure. Although infection rates are relatively low, there is a risk of developing a deep infection around the joint replacement. Prompt treatment with antibiotics is crucial if an infection occurs.

2. Blood clots

Joint replacement surgery carries a risk of developing blood clots, particularly deep vein thrombosis (DVT) in the legs. Measures are taken before, during, and after surgery to prevent blood clots, such as blood thinning medications, compression stockings, and early mobilization.

3. Implant complications

In some cases, complications related to the joint implant may arise. These can include implant loosening, dislocation, wear and tear, or fracture. While advancements in implant design and surgical techniques have reduced the occurrence of these complications, they can still happen and may require additional surgery to address.

4. Nerve or blood vessel injury

There is a small risk of damaging surrounding nerves or blood vessels during the surgical procedure. Surgeons take precautions to minimize this risk, but in some cases, nerve damage or impaired blood flow may occur, leading to numbness, weakness, or other complications.

5. Anesthesia risks

Joint replacement surgery requires anesthesia, which carries its own risks. The anesthesiologist will assess the patient's health and determine the most appropriate type of anesthesia to use, taking into consideration individual factors and potential risks.

It's important to note that the overall success of joint replacement surgery depends on various factors, including the individual's overall health, adherence to rehabilitation protocols, and active participation in post-operative care. It is essential to have open and honest discussions with the healthcare team to fully understand the benefits, risks, and expected outcomes of joint replacement surgery based on each individual's unique situation.

Arthroscopy and Joint Resurfacing Procedures

Arthroscopy and joint resurfacing procedures are two surgical techniques used in the treatment of joint conditions, including osteoarthritis.

Here's an overview of each procedure:

1. Arthroscopy

Arthroscopy is a minimally invasive surgical procedure that involves inserting a small camera, called an arthroscope, into the joint through small incisions. The arthroscope provides real-time images of the joint's interior, allowing the surgeon to diagnose and treat various joint conditions.

During arthroscopy, specialized instruments are used to address specific joint issues. These may include removing loose cartilage or bone fragments, repairing damaged tissues (such as torn ligaments or tendons), smoothing out irregular joint surfaces, or removing inflamed synovial tissue. The procedure is typically performed on larger joints such as the knee, shoulder, or hip.

Arthroscopy offers several benefits, including smaller incisions, reduced tissue trauma, shorter recovery time, and potentially less pain compared to traditional open surgery. It can help relieve symptoms, improve joint function, and delay the need for more invasive procedures like joint replacement.

2. Joint Resurfacing Procedures

Joint resurfacing procedures involve smoothing out or reshaping the damaged joint surfaces without completely replacing the joint. These procedures are often considered for individuals with localized joint damage or specific joint conditions, particularly in younger patients who may not be suitable candidates for joint replacement surgery.

The goal of joint resurfacing is to alleviate pain, improve joint function, and preserve as much of the natural joint as possible. The damaged portions of the joint surfaces are removed and replaced with metal or other materials, allowing for improved joint mechanics and reduced friction. Joint resurfacing procedures can be performed in various joints, including the hip, knee, or shoulder.

It's important to note that joint resurfacing procedures are not suitable for all individuals or all types of joint damage. The decision to pursue joint resurfacing is based on factors such as the extent and location of the joint damage, overall health, and individual considerations. The healthcare professional will assess the specific condition and determine the most appropriate course of action.

As with any surgical procedure, there are potential risks and complications associated with arthroscopy and joint resurfacing procedures. These can include infection, blood clots, nerve or blood vessel injury, and potential limitations in long-term durability. It's important to discuss these risks with the healthcare team and have a clear understanding of the expected benefits and potential drawbacks of these surgical techniques based on the individual's specific situation.

Rehabilitation and Recovery after Surgery

Rehabilitation and recovery play a crucial role in achieving optimal outcomes following orthopedic surgery, including procedures for osteoarthritis. The rehabilitation process is designed to restore joint function, promote healing, reduce pain, and improve overall mobility.

Here are some key aspects of rehabilitation and recovery after surgery:

1. Physical Therapy

Physical therapy is an essential component of rehabilitation after surgery. A physical therapist will work closely with the patient to develop a personalized exercise program aimed at restoring joint range of motion, strengthening muscles, and improving overall mobility. Physical therapy may involve various techniques such as stretching exercises, strengthening exercises, balance training, and functional movements specific to the affected joint.

2. Pain Management

Effective pain management is crucial during the recovery period. Pain medication prescribed by the healthcare team may help manage post-operative pain. Additionally, other pain management techniques such as ice or heat therapy, transcutaneous electrical nerve stimulation (TENS), and elevation of the affected joint can provide relief. It's important to follow the healthcare provider's instructions regarding pain management.

3. Wound Care

Proper wound care is essential to prevent infection and promote healing. It's important to keep the surgical incision site clean and dry as instructed by the healthcare team. They will provide specific guidelines on wound care, such as when and how to change dressings and signs of infection to watch out for.

4. Assistive Devices

Depending on the type of surgery and the joint involved, assistive devices such as crutches, walkers, or splints may be recommended to support mobility and protect the healing joint. These devices help with weight-bearing, balance, and stability during the initial stages of recovery.

5. Gradual Return to Activities

The healthcare team will provide guidance on gradually increasing activities and exercises as the healing process progresses. It's important to follow their recommendations and avoid overexertion or engaging in high-impact activities that may strain the joint. The timing and pace of returning to activities will vary depending on the specific surgical procedure and the individual's progress.

6. Follow-up Appointments

Regular follow-up appointments with the healthcare team are essential to monitor progress, address any concerns, and make necessary adjustments to the rehabilitation program. These appointments allow the healthcare team to assess the healing process, track range of motion and strength improvements, and provide guidance on the next steps in the recovery journey.

It's important to note that the duration of rehabilitation and recovery can vary depending on the type of surgery, the individual's overall health, and their commitment to following the prescribed rehabilitation program. Each person's recovery process is unique, and it's important to be patient and adhere to the recommended guidelines for a successful recovery.

During the rehabilitation period, it's also beneficial to maintain a healthy lifestyle by following a balanced diet, staying hydrated, getting adequate rest, and avoiding smoking or excessive alcohol consumption. These factors can contribute to overall healing and enhance the recovery process.

Lastly, open communication with the healthcare team is crucial throughout the rehabilitation process. If any concerns or questions arise during recovery, it's important to discuss them with the healthcare provider for appropriate guidance and support.

Chapter 11

Living a Fulfilling Life with Osteoarthritis

Living a fulfilling life with osteoarthritis is absolutely possible with the right mindset, self-care strategies, and support. While osteoarthritis may present challenges, it doesn't have to define or limit your life.

Here are some tips to help you live a fulfilling life with osteoarthritis:

1. Education and Understanding

Educate yourself about osteoarthritis, including its causes, symptoms, and treatment options. Understanding your condition can help you make informed decisions and actively participate in managing your health.

2. Positive Mindset

Adopt a positive mindset and focus on what you can do rather than what you can't. Accepting and adapting to the changes imposed by osteoarthritis is key to maintaining a fulfilling life. Embrace a resilient attitude and stay optimistic about the possibilities that lie ahead.

3. Self-Care and Healthy Lifestyle

Prioritize self-care and maintain a healthy lifestyle. This includes eating a balanced diet, engaging in regular physical activity (with modifications as needed), getting sufficient rest and sleep, managing stress through relaxation techniques or hobbies, and avoiding smoking and excessive alcohol consumption. Taking care of your overall well-being can positively impact your ability to manage osteoarthritis and maintain a fulfilling life.

4. Physical Activity and Exercise

Stay physically active within the limits of your condition. Regular exercise can help strengthen muscles, improve joint flexibility and mobility, and manage weight, all of which can alleviate symptoms and enhance your quality of life. Consult with your healthcare team or a physical therapist to develop an exercise program tailored to your specific needs and abilities.

5. Pain Management

Develop effective pain management strategies in consultation with your healthcare team. This may include a combination of medication, heat or cold therapy, gentle stretching exercises, relaxation techniques, and using assistive devices to minimize joint stress. Communicate openly with your healthcare provider to find the best approach for managing your pain.

6. Support Network

Surround yourself with a strong support network of family, friends, and healthcare professionals who understand and empathize with your experience. Share your challenges, seek advice and encouragement, and lean on their support during difficult times. Consider joining support groups or online communities where you can connect with others who are going through similar experiences.

7. Adaptations and Assistive Devices

Explore adaptations and assistive devices that can help you perform daily activities more easily. This may include using ergonomic tools, assistive devices for walking or gripping, or modifying your living environment to reduce joint strain and increase accessibility. Occupational therapists can provide valuable guidance on making necessary adaptations.

8. Pursue Hobbies and Interests

Engage in activities that bring you joy and fulfillment. Pursue hobbies, interests, and creative outlets that are compatible with your abilities. Whether it's gardening, painting, playing a musical instrument, or exploring new hobbies, focusing on activities that inspire and uplift you can help maintain a sense of purpose and fulfillment.

9. Emotional Well-being

Pay attention to your emotional well-being and seek support when needed. Living with chronic pain can sometimes lead to emotional challenges such as anxiety or depression. Consider seeking professional counseling or therapy to help navigate these emotions and develop coping strategies.

Remember, living a fulfilling life with osteoarthritis is about embracing your abilities, making necessary adaptations, and focusing on what brings you joy and purpose. Each person's journey is unique, so it's important to tailor these suggestions to your specific needs and preferences. Consult with your healthcare team for personalized advice and guidance as you navigate your life with osteoarthritis.

Strategies for Managing Flare-Ups

Flare-ups in osteoarthritis refer to episodes of increased pain, inflammation, and other symptoms that are typically temporary and occur periodically. They can be characterized by a sudden worsening of joint pain, stiffness, swelling, and reduced joint function. Flare-ups can vary in intensity and duration, ranging from mild and short-lived to more severe and lasting for several days or weeks.

Several factors can contribute to the occurrence of flare-ups in osteoarthritis:

1. Joint Overuse or Injury

Engaging in excessive physical activity, repetitive motions, or placing excessive stress on the affected joints can trigger a flare-up. Activities such as heavy lifting, prolonged standing, or repetitive joint movements can exacerbate symptoms.

2. Joint Inflammation

Osteoarthritis involves inflammation in the affected joints. Flare-ups can occur when this inflammation becomes more pronounced, leading to increased pain, swelling, and stiffness.

3. Weather Changes

Some individuals with osteoarthritis may notice an increase in symptoms during changes in weather, particularly in cold and damp conditions. The exact reasons behind this association are not fully understood, but changes in barometric pressure and temperature might play a role.

4. Infection or Injury

Joint infections or injuries, even minor ones, can trigger a flare-up of osteoarthritis symptoms. These events can cause an inflammatory response in the joint, leading to increased pain and discomfort.

5. Lifestyle Factors

Certain lifestyle factors, such as stress, lack of sleep, poor nutrition, and excessive weight, can contribute to the frequency and severity of flare-ups. Managing these factors through healthy habits and self-care strategies can help minimize the occurrence of flare-ups.

Managing flare-ups in osteoarthritis involves a combination of self-care strategies, medication, and other treatments to alleviate symptoms and promote healing. Resting the affected joint, applying heat or cold therapy, taking over-the-counter pain relievers, and practicing gentle exercises or physical therapy can help manage flare-ups.

It's essential to work closely with a healthcare provider to develop an individualized treatment plan that addresses your specific needs and helps you effectively manage flare-ups as they occur.

Flare-ups of osteoarthritis can be challenging to manage, but there are strategies that can help alleviate symptoms and minimize their impact on your daily life.

Here are some strategies for managing flare-ups:

1. Rest and Protect the Joint

During a flare-up, it's important to give the affected joint adequate rest. Avoid activities that exacerbate pain or put excessive strain on the joint. Use assistive devices, such as crutches or braces, if necessary, to protect the joint and reduce weight-bearing.

2. Apply Heat or Cold Therapy

Applying heat or cold therapy can help relieve pain and reduce inflammation during a flare-up. Heat therapy, such as warm compresses or heating pads, can help relax muscles and promote blood flow. Cold therapy, such as ice packs or cold compresses, can numb the area and reduce swelling. Experiment with both heat and cold to see which works best for you.

3. Medications

Over-the-counter pain relievers, such as acetaminophen or nonsteroidal anti-inflammatory drugs (NSAIDs), can help manage pain and reduce inflammation. Consult with your healthcare provider for guidance on the appropriate medications and dosages for your specific situation. It's important to use medications as directed and be aware of potential side effects.

4. Gentle Exercises and Stretching

While rest is important, gentle exercises and stretching can help maintain joint flexibility and mobility during a flare-up. Low-impact activities, such as swimming or walking in water, gentle range-of-motion exercises, and stretching can help reduce stiffness and improve joint function. Consult with a physical therapist for guidance on exercises that are safe and appropriate for your condition.

5. Joint Protection Techniques

Practice joint protection techniques to minimize stress on the affected joint. This includes using proper body mechanics during daily activities, avoiding repetitive motions, lifting and carrying objects correctly, and using assistive devices or adaptive equipment to reduce joint strain.

6. Weight Management

Maintaining a healthy weight can help reduce the load on your joints, which can alleviate symptoms during flare-ups. If necessary, consult with a registered dietitian or healthcare provider to develop a weight management plan that suits your needs.

7. Stress Management

Flare-ups can be stressful both physically and emotionally. Stress can exacerbate pain and inflammation, so it's important to find effective stress management techniques. This may include practicing relaxation techniques, such as deep breathing exercises, meditation, or engaging in activities that help you unwind and reduce stress levels.

8. Support Network

Reach out to your support network, including family, friends, or support groups, during flare-ups. Sharing your experience, seeking understanding, and getting emotional support can make a significant difference in coping with flare-ups.

9. Communication with Healthcare Provider

Keep an open line of communication with your healthcare provider. Inform them about your flare-ups, symptoms, and any changes you experience. They can provide guidance, adjust your treatment plan if necessary, and offer recommendations for managing flare-ups effectively.

Remember, everyone's experience with flare-ups is unique, and it may take time to find the strategies that work best for you. Be patient and persistent in exploring different techniques and seeking professional guidance as needed.

Balancing Activity and Rest

Balancing activity and rest is crucial for managing osteoarthritis and preventing flare-ups. Finding the right balance can help maintain joint health, manage symptoms, and preserve overall function.

Here are some strategies for achieving a healthy balance between activity and rest:

1. Listen to Your Body

Pay close attention to how your body feels during and after physical activity. If you experience increased pain, swelling, or joint discomfort, it may be a sign that you need to modify your activity level or take a rest. Respect your body's signals and adjust your activities accordingly.

2. Gradual Progression

When starting or increasing physical activity, do it gradually. Gradual progression allows your body to adapt and adjust to the demands placed on the joints. Begin with low-impact exercises and gradually increase the intensity or duration over time. This approach can help minimize the risk of overexertion and potential flare-ups.

3. Low-Impact Exercise

Engage in low-impact exercises that are gentle on the joints, such as swimming, water aerobics, stationary biking, or walking on soft surfaces. These activities provide cardiovascular benefits, improve joint mobility, and strengthen the surrounding muscles without placing excessive stress on the joints.

4. Range-of-Motion Exercises

Incorporate regular range-of-motion exercises to maintain joint flexibility. These exercises help improve joint mobility, reduce stiffness, and prevent joint contractures. Gentle stretching and activities that promote joint movement, such as yoga or tai chi, can be beneficial.

5. Strength Training

Include strength training exercises in your routine to strengthen the muscles around the affected joints. Strong muscles provide better joint support and can help alleviate stress on the joints. Work with a physical therapist or a qualified fitness professional to develop a safe and effective strength training program.

6. Rest and Recovery

Allow yourself adequate time for rest and recovery between activities. This includes scheduled rest days in your exercise routine and taking breaks during activities that require prolonged joint use. Listen to your body's need for rest and give yourself permission to take breaks when necessary.

7. Joint Protection Techniques

Practice joint protection techniques to minimize stress on the affected joints during daily activities. This includes using proper body mechanics, avoiding repetitive movements, and using assistive devices or adaptive equipment to reduce joint strain.

8. Individualize Your Approach

Remember that each person's capabilities and limitations may vary. What works for someone else may not work for you. Pay attention to your unique needs, limitations, and comfort levels. Consult with healthcare professionals, such as physical therapists or occupational therapists, who can provide personalized guidance and recommendations based on your specific condition.

By striking a balance between activity and rest, you can maintain joint health, manage symptoms, and enhance your overall well-being with osteoarthritis. Listen to your body, be mindful of your limitations, and make adjustments as needed to achieve a balanced and sustainable approach to physical activity and rest.

Setting Realistic Goals and Expectations

Setting realistic goals and expectations is an important aspect of managing osteoarthritis and maintaining emotional well-being. When living with a chronic condition like osteoarthritis, it's crucial to have achievable goals and realistic expectations to avoid disappointment, frustration, and potential setbacks.

Here are some strategies for setting realistic goals and expectations:

1. Understand Your Condition

Educate yourself about osteoarthritis, including its symptoms, progression, and treatment options. This knowledge will help you gain a realistic understanding of what to expect and what limitations you may face. Consult with healthcare professionals who can provide accurate information and guidance.

2. Focus on Function and Quality of Life

Instead of solely focusing on eliminating pain or achieving perfect joint function, shift your focus to improving your overall function and quality of life. Set goals that are specific, measurable, attainable, relevant, and time-bound (SMART goals) that align with your priorities and values.

3. Start Small and Gradually Progress

Break down large goals into smaller, manageable steps. By taking gradual steps and celebrating small victories, you can build momentum, maintain motivation, and see steady progress. Remember that progress may be slow and vary from person to person.

4. Be Realistic about Limitations

Recognize and accept your physical limitations. Understand that there may be activities or movements that are no longer feasible or may require modifications. Adjust your goals and expectations to align with your current abilities, ensuring you don't push yourself beyond your limits and risk exacerbating symptoms.

5. Consult with Healthcare Professionals

Work closely with your healthcare team, including doctors, physical therapists, and occupational therapists, to set realistic goals and develop a personalized treatment plan. They can provide guidance on appropriate exercises, lifestyle modifications, and assistive devices that can help you reach your goals safely and effectively.

6. Embrace Flexibility

Osteoarthritis symptoms can fluctuate, and there may be periods of improvement and times when symptoms worsen. Be prepared to adjust your goals and expectations based on your current health status. Embracing flexibility allows you to adapt to changing circumstances and avoid feeling discouraged when setbacks occur.

7. Celebrate Progress and Practice Self-Compassion

Acknowledge and celebrate your achievements, no matter how small they may seem. Recognize the effort you put into managing your condition and making positive changes. Be kind to yourself and practice self-compassion, understanding that living with osteoarthritis can be challenging at times.

8. Seek Support

Surround yourself with a supportive network, including family, friends, or support groups. They can provide encouragement, understanding, and practical assistance as you work towards your goals. Sharing experiences and challenges with others who have similar conditions can be helpful in managing expectations.

By setting realistic goals and expectations, you can maintain a positive outlook, reduce stress, and enhance your ability to cope with the challenges of osteoarthritis. Remember that everyone's journey is unique, and it's important to focus on your individual progress and well-being.

Chapter 12

Empowering Yourself in the Osteoarthritis Journey

Empowering yourself in the osteoarthritis journey is an essential aspect of managing the condition and improving your overall well-being. It involves taking an active role in your care, making informed decisions, and advocating for your needs. By becoming an empowered individual, you can navigate the challenges of osteoarthritis with confidence and improve your quality of life.

Education is a key component of empowerment. Take the initiative to educate yourself about osteoarthritis by learning about its causes, symptoms, and available treatment options. Stay updated on the latest research and medical advancements in the field. This knowledge will enable you to have informed discussions with healthcare professionals, ask relevant questions, and actively participate in your care decisions.

Effective communication with your healthcare team is crucial. Establish open and honest lines of communication, express your concerns, and ask for clarification when needed. Actively engage in discussions about your treatment plan and collaborate with your healthcare professionals to develop a care approach that suits your specific needs and goals.

Self-management is another important aspect of empowerment. Take responsibility for managing your osteoarthritis by adopting healthy lifestyle habits. Engage in regular exercise to strengthen your muscles and joints, follow a balanced diet to support overall health, maintain a healthy weight to reduce joint stress, manage stress levels, and prioritize rest and relaxation. By actively participating in self-management, you can improve your symptoms and enhance your well-being.

Seeking support is vital in the osteoarthritis journey. Connect with support groups, online communities, or organizations dedicated to osteoarthritis. Interacting with others who share similar experiences can provide emotional support, practical advice, and a sense of belonging. Sharing your own journey and learning from others can be empowering and inspiring.

Advocacy plays a significant role in empowering yourself. Be an active advocate for your own needs and preferences in healthcare settings. Clearly communicate your concerns, treatment preferences, and goals to your healthcare team. If necessary, seek a second opinion to ensure you are receiving the best possible care. Stand up for your rights as a patient and actively participate in decision-making processes related to your treatment and management.

Taking care of your overall well-being is an essential part of empowerment. Practice self-care activities that promote physical, mental, and emotional health. Engage in activities that bring you joy and fulfillment, pursue hobbies and interests, practice relaxation techniques, and seek counseling or therapy if needed. Nurturing yourself holistically empowers you to better manage the challenges of osteoarthritis and maintain a positive outlook.

Finally, maintain a positive mindset and develop resilience. Focus on the things you can control, adapt to challenges, and find ways to overcome obstacles. Surround yourself with supportive and positive influences that uplift and encourage you on your osteoarthritis journey.

By empowering yourself, you can actively participate in your care, make informed decisions, and enhance your overall well-being. Remember that empowerment is a continuous process, and it's important to be patient and kind to yourself along the way. With empowerment, you can navigate the challenges of osteoarthritis with confidence and live a fulfilling life.

Taking Control of Your Osteoarthritis Management

Taking control of your osteoarthritis management is crucial for effectively managing the condition and improving your quality of life. By actively participating in your care and implementing strategies to manage symptoms, you can regain a sense of control and enhance your overall well-being.

Here are some key steps to take control of your osteoarthritis management:

1. Education

Educate yourself about osteoarthritis. Learn about the causes, symptoms, and progression of the condition. Understand the available treatment options, including both medical and non-medical approaches. Stay informed about the latest research and advancements in osteoarthritis management. Knowledge empowers you to make informed decisions and actively participate in your care.

2. Communication with Healthcare Professionals

Establish a strong and open line of communication with your healthcare team. Regularly discuss your symptoms, concerns, and treatment options. Ask questions and seek clarification on any aspect of your condition or treatment plan. Collaborate with your healthcare professionals to develop a personalized management plan that aligns with your goals and preferences.

3. Self-Management

Take an active role in self-managing your osteoarthritis. Adopt healthy lifestyle habits that promote joint health, such as regular exercise, maintaining a healthy weight, eating a balanced diet, managing stress, and getting adequate rest. Follow any prescribed exercises or physical therapy programs to strengthen your muscles and improve joint function. Implement strategies to protect your joints during daily activities, such as using assistive devices or modifying your environment.

4. Pain Management

Develop effective pain management strategies to alleviate discomfort and improve your overall well-being. This may involve a combination of medication, physical therapy, heat or cold therapy, relaxation techniques, and alternative therapies like acupuncture or massage. Work closely with your healthcare team to find the most suitable pain management options for your specific needs.

5. Assistive Devices

Explore the use of assistive devices and adaptive tools to support your daily activities and reduce joint stress. These may include braces, splints, walking aids (canes or walkers), ergonomic tools, or modifications to your home or workplace. Consult with an occupational therapist or physical therapist to identify and obtain the most appropriate assistive devices for your needs.

6. Emotional Support

Seek emotional support from family, friends, support groups, or mental health professionals. Living with a chronic condition like osteoarthritis can be emotionally challenging, and having a strong support network can provide encouragement, understanding, and coping strategies. Sharing your experiences, feelings, and concerns with others who are going through similar situations can be empowering and uplifting.

7. Monitor and Track Progress

Keep track of your symptoms, treatments, and any lifestyle modifications you make. Monitor how certain activities or interventions affect your pain levels and overall well-being. This information can help you identify patterns, determine what works best for you, and make adjustments to your management plan as needed.

8. Stay Positive and Motivated

Maintain a positive mindset and stay motivated throughout your osteoarthritis management journey. Focus on the progress you make, no matter how small, and celebrate your achievements. Engage in activities that bring you joy and fulfillment, and cultivate a sense of purpose beyond your condition. Remember that managing osteoarthritis is a long-term process, and it's important to maintain a positive outlook and persevere through challenges.

Taking control of your osteoarthritis management empowers you to actively participate in your care and make informed decisions. By implementing strategies to manage symptoms, practicing self-care, seeking support, and maintaining a positive mindset, you can optimize your quality of life and effectively manage osteoarthritis. Remember to work closely with your healthcare team, stay informed, and adapt your management plan as needed to meet your evolving needs.

Looking Towards the Future with Hope and Resilience

Looking towards the future with hope and resilience is crucial when living with osteoarthritis. While the condition may present challenges and uncertainties, maintaining a positive outlook can greatly impact your overall well-being and ability to cope. Cultivating hope and resilience involves adopting strategies that empower you to face the future with optimism and strength.

One important strategy is to focus on what you can control. Osteoarthritis may bring limitations, but it's essential to concentrate on the things within your control. Take charge of your self-care by adhering to your treatment plan, practicing healthy lifestyle choices, and managing your symptoms. By focusing on actionable steps and taking proactive measures, you can empower yourself and maintain a sense of control over your well-being.

Setting realistic goals is another key aspect of looking towards the future with hope and resilience. Establish goals that are achievable and align with your abilities and circumstances. Break larger goals into smaller, manageable steps, and celebrate each milestone you reach along the way. Recognizing and appreciating your progress, no matter how small, can provide a sense of accomplishment and motivation to continue moving forward.

Practicing self-care is vital in cultivating hope and resilience. Prioritize activities that promote physical, mental, and emotional well-being. Engage in hobbies or activities that bring you joy, relaxation, and a sense of fulfillment. This might include exercise, spending quality time with loved ones, practicing mindfulness or meditation, or seeking support from a therapist or counselor. By prioritizing self-care, you are nurturing your overall well-being and building resilience to face the challenges ahead.

Staying informed and proactive is another important aspect of looking towards the future with hope. Stay up to date on the latest advancements in osteoarthritis research, treatments, and self-management techniques. Knowledge empowers you to make informed decisions about your care and treatment options. Stay engaged with your healthcare team, ask questions, and advocate for your needs. Taking an active role in your treatment can instill a sense of hope and optimism for the future.

Seeking support is a valuable strategy in cultivating hope and resilience. Surround yourself with a supportive network of family, friends, and peers who understand and validate your experiences. Joining support groups or online communities can provide a sense of belonging, as well as opportunities to share experiences, gain insights, and find encouragement. Support from others who are facing similar challenges can be a source of strength and resilience during difficult times.

Practicing resilience is essential in the face of osteoarthritis. Embrace challenges as opportunities for growth and learning. Develop coping strategies to navigate setbacks and obstacles that may arise. Focus on your strengths, past successes, and the lessons learned from difficult experiences. Embrace flexibility and adaptability in your approach to managing osteoarthritis. Resilience is a skill that can be cultivated and can help you navigate the ups and downs of living with the condition.

Maintaining a positive mindset is a powerful tool in looking towards the future with hope and resilience. Choose to see the possibilities and opportunities that lie ahead, rather than dwelling on limitations or negative thoughts. Surround yourself with positive influences, engage in positive self-talk, and practice gratitude for the blessings in your life. Cultivating a positive mindset can foster hope and resilience in the face of adversity.

If feelings of hopelessness, anxiety, or depression persist, it may be helpful to seek support from a mental health professional. They can provide guidance, coping strategies, and therapeutic interventions to help you navigate the emotional challenges associated with osteoarthritis. Remember that resilience and hope are cultivated over time, and it's important to embrace the journey, celebrate your progress, and acknowledge your strength and perseverance. By looking towards the future with hope and resilience, you can face the challenges of osteoarthritis with a positive mindset and live a fulfilling life.

Chapter 13

Preventing Osteoarthritis

While it may not be possible to completely prevent osteoarthritis, there are certain measures you can take to reduce the risk or delay the onset of the condition.

Here are some strategies that may help:

1. Maintain a healthy weight

Excess weight puts added stress on your joints, particularly on weight-bearing joints like the knees and hips. By maintaining a healthy weight, you can reduce the strain on your joints and lower the risk of developing osteoarthritis.

2. Stay physically active

Regular exercise helps to strengthen the muscles around your joints, providing them with better support. Low-impact activities like walking, swimming, cycling, and gentle stretching can improve joint flexibility and reduce the risk of osteoarthritis. However, avoid high-impact activities that may increase joint injury risk.

3. Protect your joints

Take precautions to protect your joints from injury or overuse. Use proper techniques when lifting heavy objects, avoid repetitive motions that strain your joints, and use protective gear when participating in sports or activities that carry a higher risk of joint injury.

4. Practice good posture and body mechanics

Maintaining proper posture and using ergonomic techniques when sitting, standing, and lifting can help reduce stress on your joints and minimize the risk of developing osteoarthritis.

5. Avoid excessive joint loading

Limit activities that put excessive stress on your joints, such as repetitive kneeling, squatting, or prolonged periods of standing. If these activities are necessary, take regular breaks and use knee pads or other supportive devices to reduce joint strain.

6. Eat a balanced diet

Consuming a diet rich in fruits, vegetables, whole grains, lean proteins, and healthy fats can provide the nutrients necessary to support joint health. Omega-3 fatty acids, found in fatty fish, walnuts, and flaxseeds, have been shown to have anti-inflammatory properties that may benefit joint health.

7. Be cautious with joint injuries

Promptly treat any joint injuries or sprains and follow proper rehabilitation techniques. Untreated injuries can increase the likelihood of developing osteoarthritis in the affected joint.

8. Consider joint-friendly supplements

Certain supplements, such as glucosamine and chondroitin sulfate, have been suggested to have potential benefits for joint health. Consult with your healthcare provider before starting any supplements to ensure they are safe and suitable for you.

Remember, while these strategies can help reduce the risk of osteoarthritis, they may not guarantee complete prevention. If you have concerns about osteoarthritis or joint health, it's always a good idea to consult with a healthcare professional for personalized advice.

In conclusion, optimizing life with osteoarthritis requires a multifaceted approach that encompasses effective pain management strategies and a commitment to quality living. By implementing a combination of medical interventions, lifestyle adjustments, and self-care practices, individuals with osteoarthritis can experience improved pain control, enhanced functionality, and an overall higher quality of life.

It is essential to work closely with healthcare professionals, adopt healthy habits, and seek support from loved ones and relevant resources. With determination, resilience, and a proactive mindset, individuals can navigate the challenges of osteoarthritis and embrace a fulfilling life filled with joy, purpose, and well-being.

References

www.arthritis.org

www.mayoclinic.org

www.ncbi.nlm.nih.gov/pubmed

www.niams.nih.gov